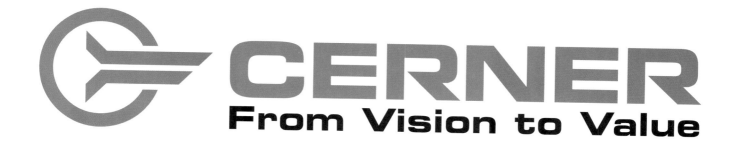

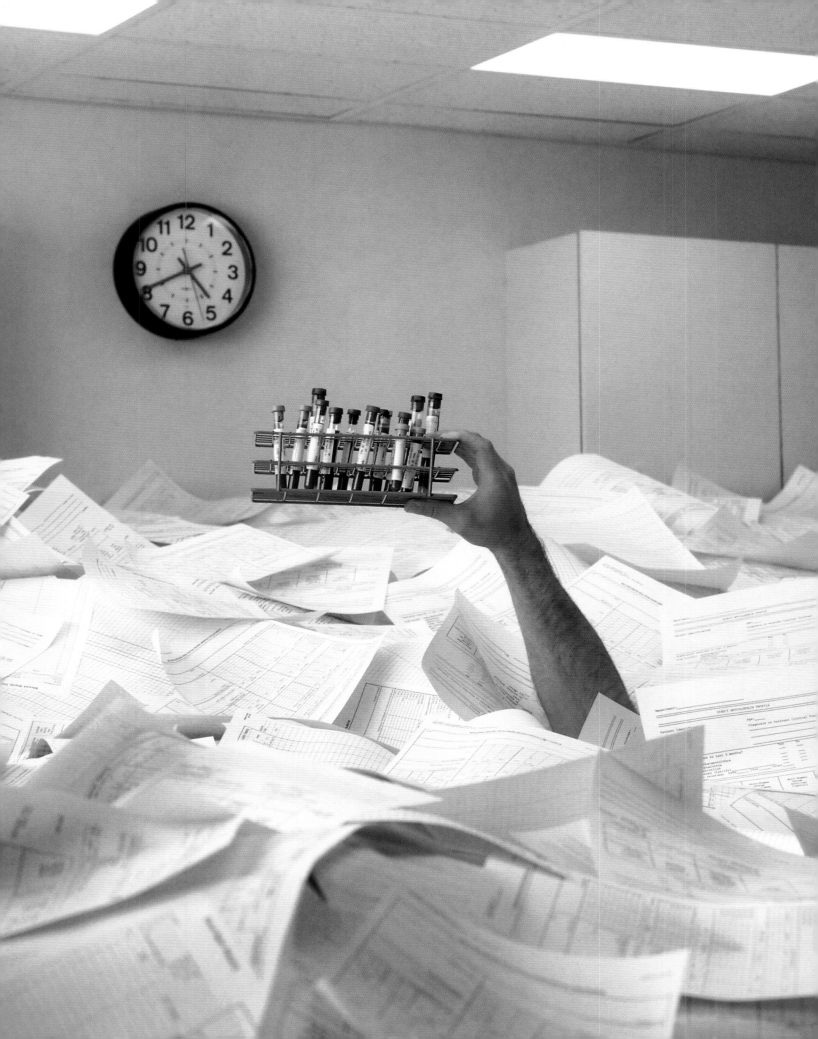

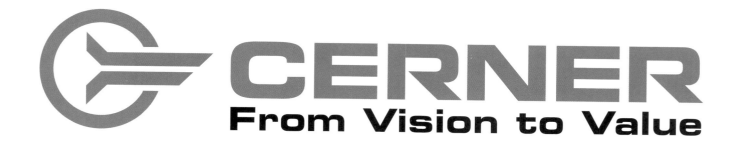

CERNER
From Vision to Value

Jeffrey L. Rodengen

Edited by Jill Gambill and Amy Blakely
Design and layout by Sandy Cruz and Rachelle Donley

Write Stuff Enterprises, Inc.
1001 South Andrews Avenue
Fort Lauderdale, FL 33316
1-800-900-Book (1-800-900-2665)
(954) 462-6657
www.writestuffbooks.com

Publisher's Cataloging-In-Publication Data
(Prepared by The Donohue Group, Inc.)

Rodengen, Jeffrey L.
    Cerner : from vision to value / Jeffrey L. Rodengen ; edited by Jill Gambill and Amy Blakely ; design and layout by Sandy Cruz and Rachelle Donley ; [foreword by John Danforth].

    p. : ill. ; cm.

    ISBN: 1-932022-11-2

    Includes bibliographical references and index.

    1. Cerner (Firm)—History. 2. Medical informatics—History. 3. Information services industry—United States—History. 4. Health services administration—Information technology—United States—History. 5. Medical records—Data processing—History. I. Gambill, Jill. II. Blakely, Amy. III. Cruz, Sandy. IV. Donley, Rachelle. V. Danforth, John C. VI. Title.

R858 .R64 2006   610/.285
                      2005932060

Also by Jeffrey L. Rodengen

The Legend of Chris-Craft

*IRON FIST:
The Lives of Carl Kiekhaefer*

*Evinrude-Johnson
and The Legend of OMC*

*Serving the Silent Service:
The Legend of Electric Boat*

The Legend of Dr Pepper/Seven-Up

The Legend of Honeywell

The Legend of Briggs & Stratton

The Legend of Ingersoll-Rand

*The Legend of Stanley:
150 Years of The Stanley Works*

The MicroAge Way

The Legend of Halliburton

The Legend of York International

The Legend of Nucor Corporation

*The Legend of Goodyear:
The First 100 Years*

The Legend of AMP

The Legend of Cessna

The Legend of VF Corporation

The Spirit of AMD

The Legend of Rowan

*New Horizons:
The Story of Ashland Inc.*

The History of American Standard

The Legend of Mercury Marine

The Legend of Federal-Mogul

*Against the Odds:
Inter-Tel—The First 30 Years*

The Legend of Pfizer

*State of the Heart:
The Practical Guide to Your Heart
and Heart Surgery*
with Larry W. Stephenson, M.D.

*The Legend of
Worthington Industries*

The Legend of IBP, Inc.

The Legend of Trinity Industries, Inc.

*The Legend of
Cornelius Vanderbilt Whitney*

The Legend of Amdahl

The Legend of Litton Industries

The Legend of Gulfstream

The Legend of Bertram
with David A. Patten

*The Legend of
Ritchie Bros. Auctioneers*

The Legend of ALLTEL
with David A. Patten

*The Yes, you can of
Invacare Corporation*
with Anthony L. Wall

*The Ship in the Balloon:
The Story of Boston Scientific
and the Development of
Less-Invasive Medicine*

The Legend of Day & Zimmermann

The Legend of Noble Drilling

Fifty Years of Innovation: Kulicke & Soffa

Biomet—From Warsaw to the World
with Richard F. Hubbard

NRA: An American Legend

The Heritage and Values of RPM, Inc.

*The Marmon Group:
The First Fifty Years*

The Legend of Grainger

The Legend of The Titan Corporation
with Richard F. Hubbard

The Legend of Discount Tire Co.
with Richard F. Hubbard

The Legend of Polaris
with Richard F. Hubbard

The Legend of La-Z-Boy
with Richard F. Hubbard

The Legend of McCarthy
with Richard F. Hubbard

InterVoice: Twenty Years of Innovation
with Richard F. Hubbard

*Jefferson-Pilot Financial:
A Century of Excellence*
with Richard F. Hubbard

The Legend of HCA
with Richard F. Hubbard

The Legend of Werner Enterprises
with Richard F. Hubbard

The History of J. F. Shea Co.
with Richard F. Hubbard

True to Our Vision
with Richard F. Hubbard

Albert Trostel & Sons
with Richard F. Hubbard

The Legend of Sovereign Bancorp
with Richard F. Hubbard

*Innovation is the Best Medicine:
the extraordinary story of Datascope*
with Richard F. Hubbard

The Legend of Guardian Industries

*The Legend of
Universal Forest Products*

*Changing the World: Polytechnic
University—The First 150 Years*

*Nothing is Impossible:
The Legend of Joe Hardy
and 84 Lumber*

*In It For The Long Haul:
The Story of CRST*

The Story of Parsons Corporation

TABLE OF CONTENTS

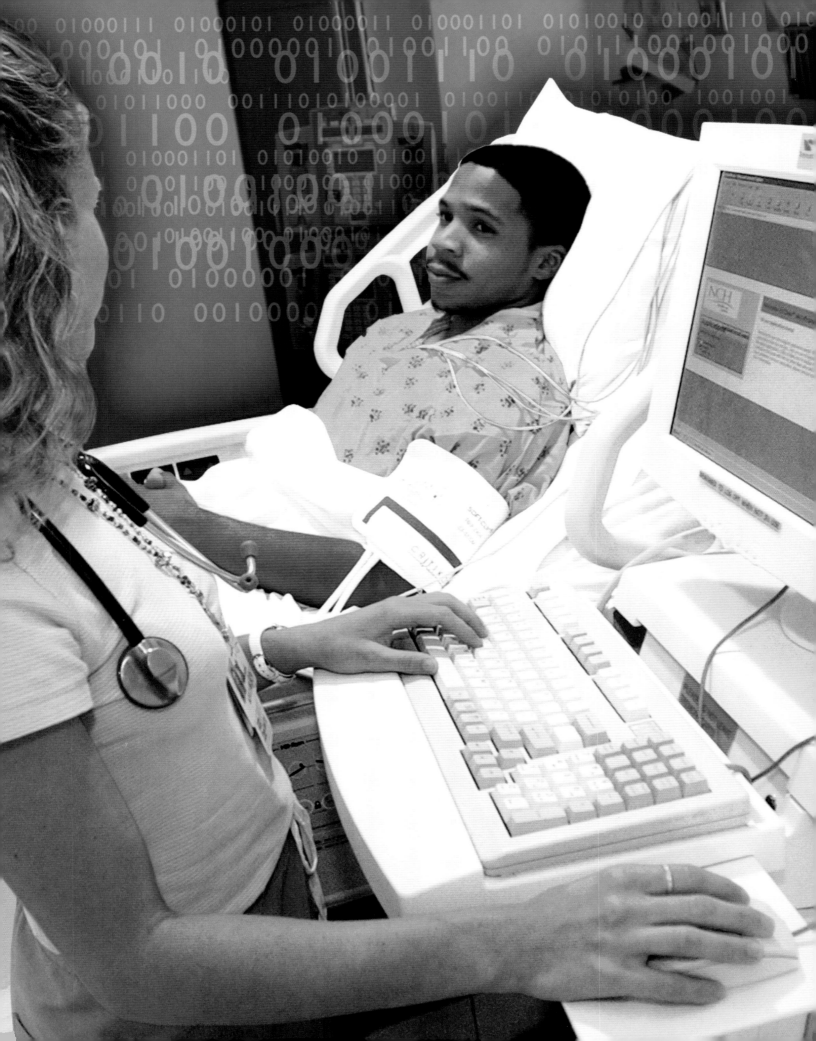

COMPANY WITH A MISSION

BY

JOHN DANFORTH

RETIRED UNITED STATES SENATOR AND
FORMER UNITED STATES AMBASSADOR TO THE UNITED NATIONS

T HE LAST TWO OF MY 18 YEARS in the United States Senate were dominated by the time-consuming, single issue of healthcare reform. We met earnestly on this subject virtually every day in one meeting or another trying to figure out how to reform healthcare. Finally, the legislative effort was so complex, and the confidence in trying to predict the effect of any legislation so minimal, that we simply could not proceed. But it was recognized that healthcare definitely had problems, and that those problems should be fixed.

One obvious problem in healthcare is that its information technology (IT) system is antiquated. There has been much mention of this. Even the President mentioned it in his State of the Union speech. It has been very well recognized that this massive industry is operating under IT standards that are lower than in other sectors of business. A consequence of healthcare's substandard IT system is the staggering rate of medical error with its tragic costs in human misery and in dollars. Much of that error can be eliminated by the effective use of software. And the most effective and efficient software is produced by *Cerner* Corporation.

Cerner and its people have as clear a vision for their company as any company I have ever known. Their mission is to reform healthcare, and that is a big vision for an industry that desperately needs to be reformed. *Cerner* is more than a business that exists for the purpose of making money, although

that's important for any business. Its mission is to make healthcare better, more efficient, more effective, more cost effective, and less prone to error.

When after 18 years in business, *Cerner* took the courageous step to design and implement an entirely new software platform of healthcare solutions, there was no guarantee of success. It was both exhilarating and nerve-wracking for those of us on the board. The new platform would eventually represent an investment of a billion dollars. It was something that the company had to do, and if *Cerner* did it, and did it well, it would lap the field. The success of *Cerner*'s new Millennium suite of software solutions established *Cerner* as being in a class by itself.

Much can be said about the passion of *Cerner* associates, both shared and generated by its founders, Neal Patterson, Cliff Illig, and Paul Gorup. Neal Patterson has said, "Healthcare is broken, and we are going to fix it." The entire organization is infused with a palpable and contagious enthusiasm to achieve the goals of making the experience of human contact with the healthcare industry more productive, less threatening, and ultimately more rewarding for patients, as well as more efficient, secure, and cost-effective for practitioners at every level.

It is indeed a very large vision, involving nothing less than leadership in the reform of healthcare. *Cerner* has accepted the challenge with great determination.

ACKNOWLEDGMENTS

A GREAT NUMBER OF people assisted in the research, preparation, and publication of *Cerner: From Vision to Value.*

The development of historical timelines and a large portion of the principal archival

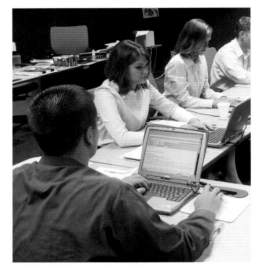

research was accomplished by research assistant Antonia Felix. Senior Editors Jill Gambill and Amy Blakely oversaw the text and photos, while the graphic design of Vice President/Creative Director Sandy Cruz brought the story to life.

The research, however, much less the book itself, would have been impossible without the dedicated assistance of *Cerner* executives and associates. Vital to this effort was the time and cooperation extended by Maria Stecklein, senior project manager, whose courteous and affable guidance made it possible for our research team to identify records and individuals crucial to *Cerner's* legacy.

Special thanks are also due to the book's review team, whose guidance in the process provided us with unique insight into *Cerner's* history: Rob Campbell, Cliff Illig, Allan Kells, April Martin, Nanette Mills, Marc Naughton, Neil Rutkowski, Randy Sims, Jeff Townsend, Don Trigg, and Julie Wilson.

All of the subjects interviewed—whether senior managers, staff, or retirees—were generous with their time and insights. Those who shared their memories and thoughts include Doug Abel, Leo Black, Paul Black, Gail Blanchard, Mike Breedlove, Dick Brown, Rob Campbell, Lupe Coursey, Alan Deitrich, Trace Devanny, Terry Dolan, Jon Doolittle, Todd Downey, John Dragovits, Bill Dwyer, J.P. Findago, Rick Fiske, Dick Flanigan, Jim Flynn, Chris Giglio, Jeff Goldsmith, Paul Gorup, Mike Herman, Matt Hodes, Rick Holbrook, Carol Hull, Cliff Illig, Bryan Ince, Gay Johannes, Allan Kells, Doug Krebs, John Kuckelman, Liane Lance, John Landis, Jay Linney, Scott MacKenzie, David McCallie, Francie McNair-Stoner, Rich Miller, Jim Mongan, Chris Murrish, Marc Naughton, Mike Neal, Steve Neubauer, Jack Newman Jr., Mike Nill, Steve Oden, Neal Patterson, Seth Rupp, Neil Rutkowski, Mark Schonhoff, Justin Scott, David Sides, Paul Sinclair, Betsy Soleburg, Jake Sorg, Shellee Spring, Owen Straub, Brian Streich, Stan Sword, Jeff Townsend, John Travis, Donald Trigg, Mike Valentine, Bill Waters, Charlotte Weaver, Julie Wilson, Matt Wilson, Janice Woods, Debbie Yantis, and Tim Zoph.

Thanks are also given to all the other associates who contributed, especially Stacey Bellomo, Colleen Belton, Rachel Boden, Dan Devers, Arch Fuston, Tricia Geris, Alicia Goforth, Shawn Kendrick, Liane Lance, Marcus Mateus, Samara Nash, and Justin Scott.

Finally, special thanks are extended to the dedicated staff at Write Stuff Enterprises, Inc.: Stanimira "Sam" Stefanova, executive editor; Ann Gossy and Mickey Murphy, senior editors; Rachelle Donley and Dennis Shockley, art directors; Bill Laznovsky, copy editor; Mary Aaron, transcriptionist; Connie Angelo, indexer; Amy Major, executive assistant to Jeffrey L. Rodengen; Marianne Roberts, executive vice president, publisher and chief financial officer; Steven Stahl, director of marketing; and Sherry Hasso, bookkeeper.

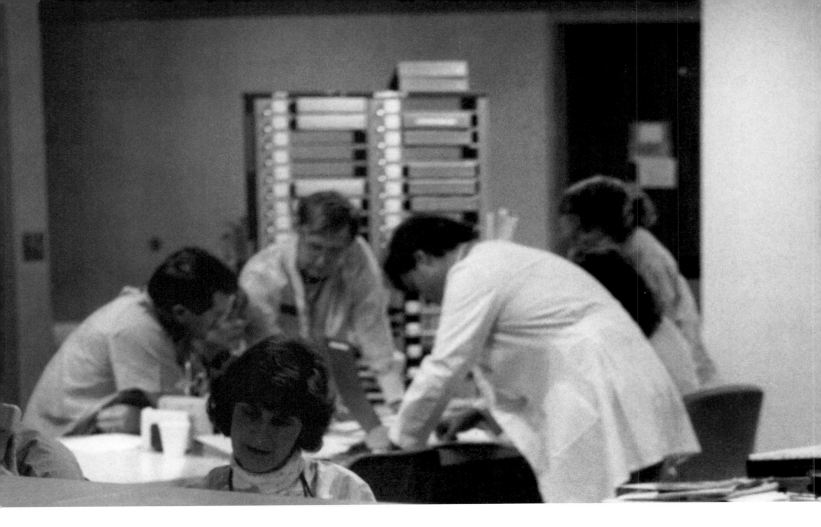

MILESTONES

1979
Neal Patterson, Paul Gorup, and Cliff Illig resign from Arthur Andersen & Co. to form their own consulting firm.

1980
Patterson, Gorup, Illig and Associates (PGI) incorporates.

1984
Company changes its name to *Cerner* Corporation.

1986
First *Cerner* Health Conference is conducted, with 35 attendees.

INTELLECTUAL PROPERTY DEVELOPMENT

1980
Development of Health Network Architecture (HNA) and *PathNet*® laboratory information system begins.

1982
PathNet® is installed in the lab at St. John Medical Center in Tulsa, Oklahoma.

1983
Company makes sales agreement with HCA, the largest hospital organization in the United States.

1984
PathNet® is introduced to the commercial marketplace.

GROWTH

1983
29 associates.

1984
Company secures first venture capital equity funding deal with First Chicago Capital Corporation for $1.5 million.

1985
Sales to Canada begin; *PathNet*® becomes available in Europe through McDonnell Douglas Corporation.

1986
Cerner goes public on Nasdaq, spend $1.085 million on *PathNet*® development.

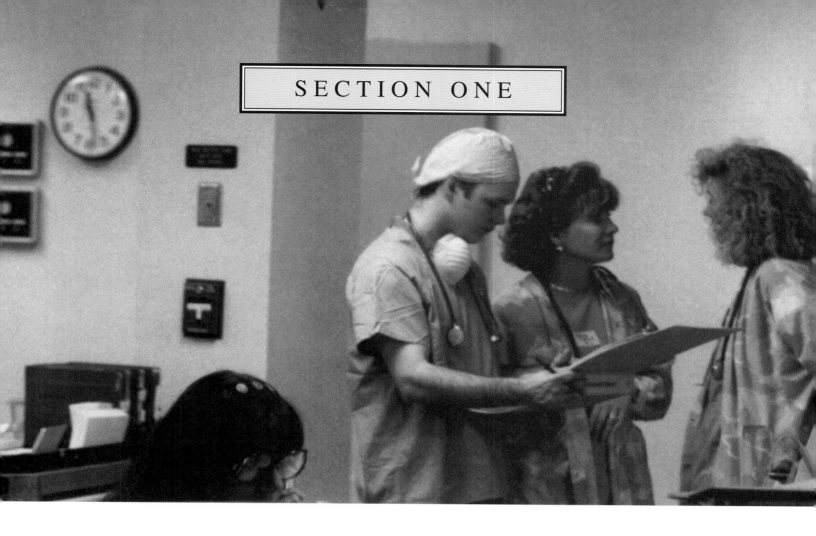

1987
Cerner is listed as one of Inc. magazine's 100 fastest-growing companies.

1989
Cerner begins participating in the Kansas City Corporate Challenge, misses first place by 0.2 points.

1990
PathNet® receives Award of Excellence from Shared Data Research.

1991
Cerner forms joint venture with El Seif Group in Saudi Arabia.

1987
MedNet®, Cerner's second solution, debuts.

1988
Cerner introduces PharmNet®, RadNet®, and Discern®.

1990
PharmNet® goes online at Washington Hospital in Washington, D.C.

1992
Cerner Vision Center opens.

1987
200 associates.

1989
Revenues amount to $56.7 million.

1991
500 associates.

1993
Revenues surpass $120 million. Branches open in Atlanta; Dallas; Boston; Irvine, California; and Washington, D.C.

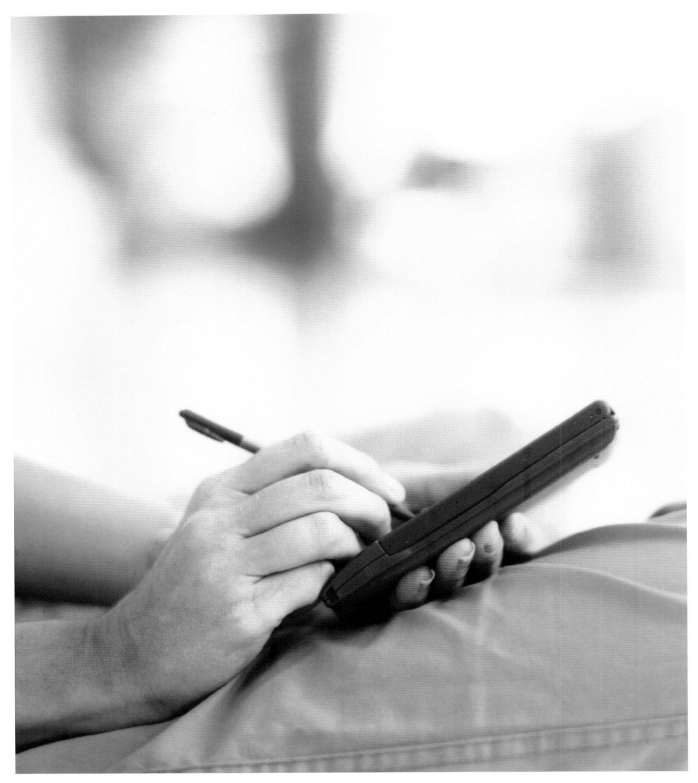

During its first 25 years, *Cerner* grew from a three-man consulting firm into a global leader in medical information technology, with nearly 7,000 associates. Its mission is to utilize technology to provide clinicians with the right information at the right time so they can make the best possible decisions for their patients. *Cerner* is taking the paper chart out of healthcare and eliminating error, variance, delay, friction, and waste in the care process.

CHAPTER ONE

ORIGINS OF INNOVATION

I believe that healthcare is fundamentally broken. Across the country, the standard of care varies, even though the science is the same and even though the biology is the same. That does not have to be the case. We have the vision and the leadership inside this company to make a major difference in how healthcare works at the core level.

—Neal Patterson,
Cerner co-founder and CEO[1]

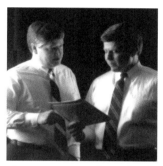

IN JUST 25 YEARS, *CERNER* Corporation has grown from a three-person consulting firm into a worldwide leader in medical information technology, with more than 1,600 clients worldwide. What began in 1979 as a picnic table brainstorming session among three young, would-be entrepreneurs has become a globally recognized corporation with nearly 7,000 associates and generating more than $1 billion a year.

Surprisingly, when the founders—Neal Patterson, Cliff Illig, and Paul Gorup—decided to establish their own consulting business, healthcare was not a target on their radar. Their list of potential clients included manufacturers, transportation companies, tax service firms, and other types of businesses. They had solid experience in those areas, while healthcare was merely a phrase scribbled on a short list of businesses that could benefit from information technology but in which they had no expertise.

Had it not been for a phone call from an overwhelmed laboratory office manager in North Kansas City, the company that became *Cerner* may have set its sights in a completely different direction.

"Can You Fix This?"

In the summer of 1979, the pathologists at MAWD—a private medical laboratory in North Kansas City named for Drs. McFee, Allen, Wright, and Dolan—couldn't understand why they didn't have any money in the bank. They did a brisk business in their office across the street from North Kansas City Hospital and by running nine other labs in town. They had hired two software designers to create a computer program to produce bills and lab reports, so they thought they had their paperwork under control.

After a lively discussion with Liane Lance, who ran their small information technology (IT) department, the doctors uncovered the source of the problem. Lance informed them that MAWD's lab manager did not trust the accuracy of the bills and had been holding on to most of them instead of mailing them out. She had been doing this for months and became completely overwhelmed as the paperwork began piling up. When Lance told the doctors about the situation, the lab manager was on vacation, and Lance decided to let them see the results for themselves.

"I took them upstairs to the lab manager's office and said, 'You need to see this,'" Lance recalled. "I opened up the cabinets and showed them months and months of bills because the manager was trying to go through them manually and correct them

Neal Patterson, right, and Cliff Illig, left, met on their first day at Arthur Andersen and became good friends while working on a project for St. Joseph Light and Power. *(Photo courtesy of © Kenny Johnson Photography.)*

AN INTRODUCTION TO *CERNER* DOCTRINES

CERNER: FROM VISION TO VALUE IS the birthplace of *Cerner* Doctrines under development today across the organization. The diverse doctrine topics range from *Cerner*'s approach to Architecture and Quality to how it performs Implementations and conducts Associate Services.

Drawing from lessons and experiences garnered throughout the company's 25-year history, straightforward principles have been developed, reflecting *Cerner*'s unique culture and methodology.

"In order to create the workforce of the future, we must capture what we've learned and reduce it to doctrine," said Cliff Illig, *Cerner* co-founder.

"We need to capture and codify our knowledge in doctrine form. Doctrines are *Cerner*'s true anthems that, taken together, differentiate us in the marketplace and the world."[1]

According to Paul Black, chief operating officer and executive vice president, "*Cerner* Doctrines represent a vision of the company and define our values, such as the concepts of treating each other with respect, taking care of our clients, and making sure that we meet the needs of the company, the shareholders, the clients, and associates."[2]

Throughout the book, key doctrine topics are highlighted upon in sidebars. Individually, each of these philosophies describe *Cerner*'s approach to...

- Architecture
- Competition
- Knowledge Management
- Managed Events
- Operational Measurement
- Quality
- Solution Development
- Vision Center

- Associate Services
- Culture
- Leadership
- Management
- Organizational Management
- Sales
- The Show

- Client Relationships
- Implementation
- Learning
- Management Implementation
- Physician Initiatives
- Service/Support
- Transformation
- Others...

manually, but she ... could never get ahead and was always working against herself."[2]

As the startled doctors gaped at the piles of paper, Lance further explained that when patients did get a bill, perhaps six months after the lab work had been performed, many of them didn't pay. They were confused by how long it had taken for the bill to show up and by the paperwork itself, which was marked up with the lab manager's corrections.[3] The payments that did come were mixed with the rest of the paperwork and had not been deposited because the office manager was hesitant to accept payment for questionable bills.

After the initial shock of seeing all their receivables hidden away in a dark corner of the lab, the

pathologists called their accountant, Tom McKittrick, for advice. He recommended they contact a young but experienced consultant who was establishing his own company and was hungry for business—Neal Patterson.

McKittrick had previously worked with Patterson, Gorup, and Illig in the Kansas City office of the accounting megafirm Arthur Andersen & Company. In the summer of 1979, Patterson had begun talking informally with Illig and Gorup about leaving the firm to start a consulting business. When McKittrick called, Patterson was still putting the group together, but he was more than happy to take a look at the lab. A potential client was just the reinforcement Patterson needed to prove

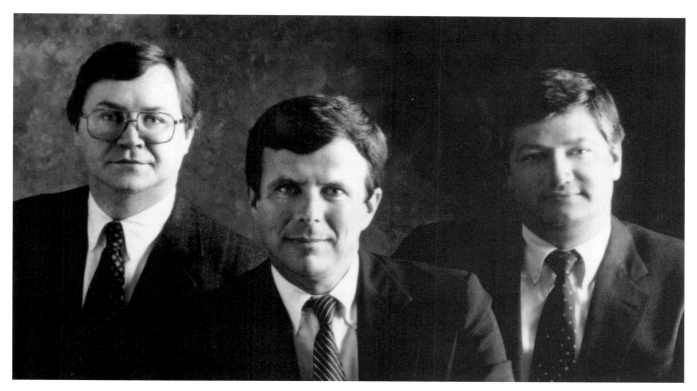

From left: Paul Gorup, Neal Patterson, and Cliff Illig resigned from Arthur Andersen in 1979 to form their own consulting company, PGI & Associates, Inc. The new firm's first clients included the MAWD laboratory, H&R Block, and Cook Paint.

to his two colleagues that there was work for them outside Andersen.

The three had talked about leaving Andersen for months, and Patterson was the first to make his move. When he finally decided to give notice, he did it so abruptly that he surprised even himself.

"I was literally walking down the hallway inside Arthur Andersen one day around the first of August, and I just decided that I would leave," he recalled. "I'd go start this business. I had not necessarily talked to Paul and Cliff about doing that. I just decided."[4]

After what he described as a "flash moment" in the hallway, Patterson walked into the office of Andersen partner Lou Wheeler and announced his resignation. "It surprised Lou a little bit," Patterson said.[5]

During his remaining four weeks at Andersen, Patterson spoke with some former Andersen asso-

ciates who had left the firm and were working in the tax and accounting services industries. "During that four weeks, I basically explored what I would go do," he said.[6]

Patterson was delighted to get the call from the struggling lab during this transition period—even though he hadn't had time to develop a fee structure or organize his new business. The pathologists were anxious to get the cash flowing and, as Patterson recalled, forced him to make some quick decisions about how he would manage his first account. As Patterson explained:

CERNER DOCTRINE

VISION

ALL CLINICAL INFORMATION SYSTEMS within a healthcare organization should interrelate to establish the foundation for high-quality, efficient patient care.

It was a very badly broken set of business processes…. So I met with them that evening, and they looked me in the eye and said, "Can you fix this?" I looked back and said with confidence, "Yes." They said, "How long will it take?" Realizing at Andersen we would have gone off and spent three weeks, four weeks preparing a proposal, I realized there was nobody to prepare a proposal…. I said it would take me three months to fix it.

They looked at me and said, "How much will it cost?" That was the one that I almost froze over, although I tried not to blink. I had no idea how to price my services. So I gave them a number, and they said they wanted to meet, which they did the next day, and they let me know they wanted me to do the work. So that was the first client.[7]

An Andersen Brotherhood

Patterson had come to Andersen fresh out of college in 1973 and had put in six years at the company before deciding to start his own consulting group. He grew up on a farm in Grant County, Oklahoma, near the small town of Manchester just south of the Kansas border. The unpredictable nature of farming taught Patterson early on about the inherent risk in every area of life—from making a living in a business dependent on something as uncontrollable as the weather, to staking his future on a new, untested vision.

"I stood out on the porch as a kid and watched a hailstorm destroy the crop," Patterson recalled. "A whole year's work … gone." But the family always bounced back from such disasters, a fact of life that also made a deep impression on Patterson. "Even though you're devastated, you know you'll still live," he said.[8]

Learning how to work through failure helped shape the proactive, risk-taking style of Neal Patterson, who became *Cerner*'s CEO.

The Pattersons were tenant farmers, and Neal and his two brothers earned money to pay for their cars and their college tuition by raising pigs on the farm.[9]

Patterson stayed close to his roots by attending Oklahoma State University in Stillwater, about 100 miles away from home. As treasurer of OSU's chapter of the Pi Kappa Alpha fraternity, Patterson displayed the business acumen that would later enable him to rise to the top tier of leadership in the healthcare industry. It was a difficult time financially for the fraternity, which had lost its house in a fire the year Patterson became a freshman. The pressure intensified as membership declined and bills went unpaid, but Patterson proved he was fit for the challenge. He managed to satisfy creditors and helped carry out a successful long-term plan to build up membership and find a new home for the chapter.[10]

Patterson earned a bachelor's degree in finance in 1971 and, one year later, an MBA. In 1973, with

A feed mill, left, and Main Street in Manchester, Oklahoma, right, near the farm in Grant County where Neal Patterson grew up.

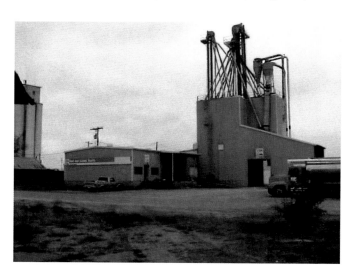
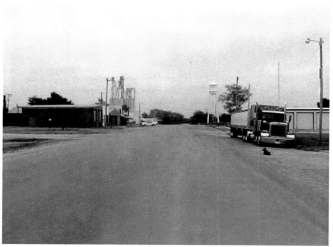

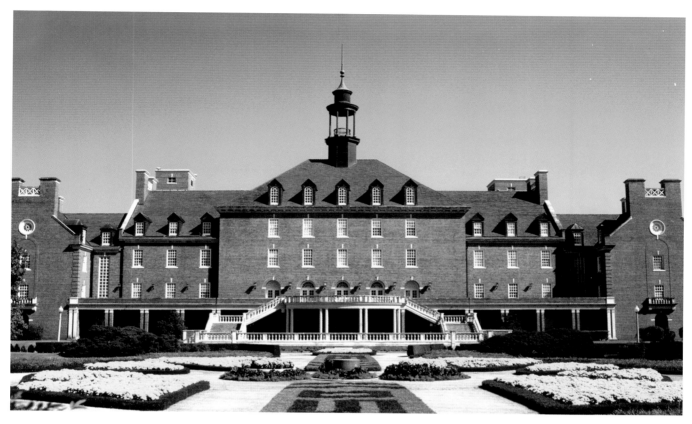

The student union at Oklahoma State University in Stillwater, where Neal Patterson earned a bachelor's degree in finance in 1971 and an MBA a year later. *(Photo courtesy of Oklahoma State University.)*

a new job as an information system consultant at Andersen, he left Oklahoma for the big city and began helping a wide range of businesses improve their bottom line.

"In the consulting division of Andersen in Kansas City, the office was small enough that the individuals weren't really specialized," said Rick Fiske, another former Andersen consultant who worked with Patterson at that time and joined *Cerner* in the mid-1980s. "We were jacks-of-all-trades in a sense—manufacturing, distribution, process management. We all had to move in and out of the industries quickly and just learn how to listen well and deal with a client to solve a business problem."[11]

Healthcare had not come up on Patterson's agenda at Andersen, however. His visit to the MAWD lab in 1979 was his first exposure to the industry, and he immediately saw the need for IT in this critical area.

Like Patterson, Illig began his career at Andersen, where he was named a system consultant, after graduating from the University of Kansas with degrees in accounting and business administration. He grew up in Kansas City, where, according to one of his Boy

Scout troop leaders, he showed early signs of being a natural entrepreneur.

"Cliff brought a set of markers down to Scout camp, and in the course of events, he would take a T-shirt, which the boy supplied, and put any design on it that he wanted," Chuck Hoffman said. "He would sketch [on] it ... with the Magic Marker™ colors, and then he got so busy that he had subcontracts going out with other kids doing the fill-in work."[12]

Both Illig and Patterson were among the small number of boys across the nation who became Eagle Scouts, and both fondly recall the life lessons that this achievement brought them.

"I remember distinctly some of the role models that were the Scout leaders of my youth," said Illig. "Scouting was ... my first exposure to results-oriented achievement."[13]

Patterson agreed. "I think fundamentally, the principles of Scouting—character and values, the Scout oath, and Scout law—they're meaningful to kids, and frankly, they've become more meaningful as I've grown up," he said.[14]

Patterson and Illig met when they started working at Andersen on the same day. "We were in the staff room and didn't know anybody to go to lunch with," Patterson recalled.[15] That day, the two men formed a lasting connection and soon found themselves working together on a project for St. Joseph Light and Power Company, a Missouri utility.

Gorup was also a recent college grad who had been hired by Arthur Andersen right out of college. Another native of Kansas City, Gorup earned an undergraduate degree in mathematics from the University of Kansas and went on to Dartmouth to earn an MBA from the university's Amos Tuck School of Business.

It took a renowned school like Tuck, famous as the first business school of its kind when it was established in 1900, to compel Gorup to leave the Midwest for New Hampshire. Gorup had always known he would follow in his father's footsteps by going into business.

His father owned a store in Kansas City that sold furniture, appliances, and electronics,[16] and Gorup grew up surrounded by all the challenges and rewards of operating a business. Although he enjoyed solving business problems for major companies at Andersen, it was only natural that at some point he would venture out on his own as his father had.

In the meantime, an Andersen job for Kansas Power and Light demanded several trips from Kansas City to Topeka every week, and Patterson and Gorup got to know each other well during those drives through the Kansas countryside.

Thorough Training

Patterson, Illig, and Gorup were all part of Andersen's Information Technology Group and underwent a computer training program required during the first two to three years on the job. The first segment was a six-week, in-house course in Programming Fundamentals, which introduced the programming language IBM Assembler. The course continued with a three-week visit to Andersen's training facility in St. Charles, Illinois, where the

student-consultants completed and tested an entire design.

"The purpose of the school was not only to teach Assembler but also to put you under pressure to meet a fixed deadline and observe how you handled the pressure," Fiske said.[17]

Back in Kansas City, the second course consisted of instruction in COBOL, followed by an initial programming assignment. Later, the consultants returned to St. Charles to learn Andersen's methodology for installing systems, as well as the company's documentation process. In the second or third year, consultants attended System Design School, which built upon previous training by expanding into the planning and design phases of a business systems development project.

Andersen's well-developed and highly structured training program created a standard set of skills that united consultants, regardless of the types of businesses they were focused upon.

"Since everyone went through the same training at roughly the same time in their career, it was reasonably easy to staff projects," Fiske said. "Everyone knew the methodology, the work papers, how to fill them out, and how a design or installation project worked. We were all trained to do the same thing, the same way, using the same tools."[18]

In its early years, *Cerner* operated in a very similar manner to Andersen. The young company's founders recruited several associates from Andersen, and the Andersen method permeated the new business.

"It's no great revelation that our installing process, work papers, etc., looked a lot like what we had been using [at Andersen]," Fiske said. "They were developed at *Cerner*, but we all were trained in the same methodology, and it showed in our approach and documentation."[19]

Brainstorming

In 1978, the three Andersen colleagues who by now had become good friends decided to flex their executive muscles by studying for the CPA exam. Bright, ambitious, and competitive, they welcomed the challenge of the notoriously difficult exam.

"Being at Andersen, even though we were on the consulting side, we thought it would be cool to prove to our accounting brethren that we all knew a fair amount about accounting," Patterson said.[20]

While studying together after working hours, the seeds for *Cerner* were planted as the consultants began to share ideas about what sort of business they could form on their own.

"It was during the preparation for that exam [that] we brainstormed the notion of 'What if we were to go create a company?' "[21] Patterson remembered. At lunch breaks during their Saturday test preparation classes, the three continued to discuss bringing their experience to a business of their own.

"I remember one lunch in which we started talking about if we weren't doing what we were doing, what would we do, and the notion of starting a business came out of that," Illig said. "It was just one of those free-flowing, fast conversations."[22]

The men had all earned reputations at Andersen as high performers, Illig added, and were therefore confident in their strengths.[23]

By now, the prep class conversations had evolved into more serious discussions on Sunday mornings around a picnic table at Kansas City's Loose Park. Illig recalled that these informal meetings, now part of *Cerner* lore, provided a relaxed setting in which to envision their ideal company:

The idea for *Cerner* was born when Patterson, Illig, and Gorup began meeting on Sunday mornings around a picnic table at Kansas City's Loose Park.

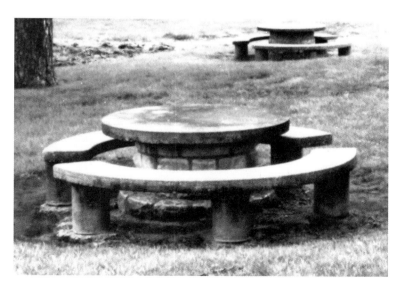

Usually these were beautiful Sunday mornings, as I recall, and cool, and we'd sit there and make lists. We had yellow spreadsheet paper. We made lists of things we were good at, things we weren't necessarily good at, of businesses we liked. We made lists of our strengths, our weaknesses. We made lists of businesses we'd seen other people leave Andersen and go into. It was out of that that we introduced the notion of being a software company. As we were working in the Andersen environment, we were watching the birth of the software industry. Why wouldn't we take what we were really good at, which was solving big business problems with information technology, and package it and find some industry to sell that to? [24]

Through their discussions, *Cerner*'s founders discovered that all three of them believed there would be great opportunity in the burgeoning software industry. The list of businesses in which they had experience—public utilities, manufacturing, distribution, transportation, entertainment, and others—far overshadowed their no-experience list, which included healthcare. They assumed that they would design systems for the industries they knew best, but the MAWD lab client—their very first—demonstrated that opportunities don't necessarily fit into neat, preconceived categories.

Patterson said, "One of the business lessons I learned fairly early is that you can create a plan and aim yourself in an area, but you have to be absolutely prepared for whatever comes because you can't predict where all the opportunity is going to come from. Opportunity is going to come from everywhere."[25]

Starting Out

In the spring of 1979, the three consultants passed the CPA exam. The weekend brainstorming sessions at Loose Park continued and culminated in Patterson's early August announcement that he was resigning from Andersen. On September 4, 1979, the firm gave Patterson its traditional send-off lunch for managers who were moving on. Patterson received some ribbing that afternoon over his newly hatched plan to start his own consulting business.

He recalled, "They were pretty much yucking this Patterson Associates, asking me, 'Who are the associates?' and 'What are you really going to go do,

THE MOST DANGEROUS MEDICAL DEVICE: THE PEN?

MEDICAL ERRORS, ACCORDING TO A report released in 1999, account for 44,000 to 98,000 deaths a year in the United States. One source of these errors is illegible physician handwriting, which results in nurses misinterpreting orders and pharmacists filling wrong prescriptions.

Cerner CEO Neal Patterson often holds up a pen when talking about the dangers of written orders and the traditional medical record. He says that when the medical industry automates its systems and eliminates the paper record, "the most dangerous medical device will be rendered useless. Without any paper, the pen will be retired."[1]

In addition to helping reduce medical errors, information technology helps eliminate the waste that permeates healthcare delivery. Integrated information technology (IT) systems cut down on duplication, such as multiple medical history forms for each person and the same tests being ordered more than once.

The healthcare consumer also is better served with an electronic medical record that can be accessed at any time by any caregiver, in contrast to a paper folder that can only be read by one practitioner at a time and has to be physically transported between departments.

Adopting IT systems also reduces the time doctors and other clinicians spend on paperwork. The American Hospital Association estimates that clinicians spend 30 to 60 minutes completing paperwork for each hour of patient care.[2] This not only reduces the time available for doctor-patient contact, but also limits the number of patients a doctor can see each day.

Even though conversion to automated systems has been slow, each year—as evidenced by the extraordinary growth of *Cerner*—more healthcare providers invest in medical IT to eliminate longstanding problems and improve the quality of care at every level.

Neal?' I'm pretty sure they thought I was crazy and that I would starve to death or would soon be back either working for somebody or begging for a job back at Andersen."[26]

But the night before, Patterson had convinced Illig and Gorup that now was the time to resign from Andersen to become the "associates" in his new startup. He had already lined up some work and was adamant that there were many more businesses that would jump at the chance to obtain their expert services at good rates. His enthusiasm hit home.

"It had been a good week," Patterson said. "I had sold more work than one person could do alone."[27]

Andersen's managers were surprised, at the very least, to learn that three of their top consultants were leaving to join Patterson's company within the space of one week.

"From the lunch, they all went back to their offices, and it was that afternoon that Cliff and Paul both resigned to create what turned out to be called Patterson, Gorup, Illig & Associates, Inc.," Patterson said. "Within one week, the three of us were out of the firm and have never looked back since."[28]

The arrangement of the founders' initials was altered slightly to avoid an awkward acronym that the founders knew they would never live down. "On September 11th, 'P' was joined by 'I' and 'G,' " Patterson said. "Our next big decision was to name our new firm PGI rather than P.I.G."[29]

Later that month, the group rented space in a building on Madison Avenue in the Plaza section of

Kansas City, and PGI incorporated a few months later in 1980. The excellent working relationships they had developed with clients over the years at Andersen helped them collect a solid client list within the first weeks. Cook Paint, a paint and varnish company headquartered in Kansas City that all three founders had worked with while at Andersen, and H&R Block were eager to retain the services of consultants they had come to trust and depend upon.

"They made the point that they were counting on us, not just Andersen, and actually created for us a fairly profitable consulting business pretty quickly," Illig said.[30]

Patterson added that he had been careful about not talking to these clients before leaving the firm and was therefore "not competing directly against Andersen."[31]

Patterson's first job was to fix the MAWD laboratory billing fiasco. As promised, he

Right: Neal Patterson encountered future *Cerner* executive Liane Lance when she was a young medical technologist at the MAWD laboratory in North Kansas City.

Below: The IBM129 punch card machine was the main component of the medical IT department at MAWD when the lab became PGI & Associates' first client in 1979. *(Photo courtesy of Bolo's Computer Museum — www.bolo.ch)*

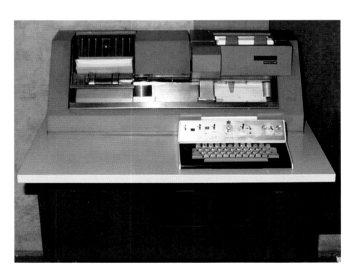

completed the task in three months. First, he gathered all the payments that were interspersed among the bills and deposited them. "This helped the bank account a lot," he noted. The rest of the work was so massive that he used a yardstick to measure his progress. Stacks of bills neatly organized into 15 work stations inched their way lower and lower as the work advanced, and Patterson made note of how many inches of paperwork the consultants sorted out every day.[32]

The MAWD project also introduced Patterson to a young computer programmer/medical technician who would eventually design *Cerner*'s first laboratory solution, *PathNet®*. Liane Lance, who ran MAWD's computer department, made a big impression on Patterson on his first visit to the lab.

"You could tell from the moment you walked in that Liane was someone—even though she was very young—who was the leader of the group, and to whom people, including the pathologists, would turn for solutions to their problems."[33]

Dr. Earl Wright had hired Lance from North Kansas City Hospital, where she had been working in the lab as a phlebotomist. In addition to assigning her med-tech duties at MAWD, Wright sent her to school to learn computer programming and subsequently put her in charge of the lab's new IT department. Wright knew that Lance's rare combination of a med-tech and computer science background would be a great asset to Patterson in creating a better billing system.

"Within less than a month," Lance recalled, "Earl Wright pulled me aside and said, 'You work for this guy. However he needs you to help, help him.' That was how Neal got exposed to the clinical setting."[34]

The founders would later marvel at the presage of this first project. *Cerner* would go on to develop groundbreaking systems to help clinicians organize and access medical data, launching the firm ahead of the pack of other hospital software companies that primarily focused on billing and other administrative applications.

The real promise of technology in healthcare, the founders soon came to believe, lay in automating complex functions and connecting fragmented hospital systems. Billing was a relatively simple,

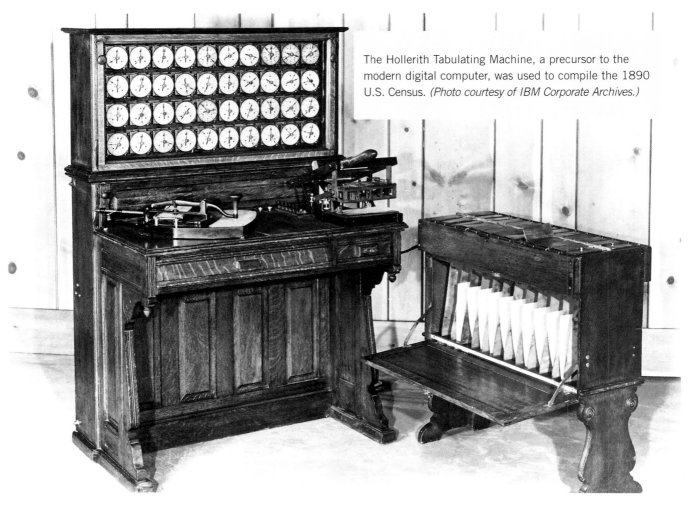

The Hollerith Tabulating Machine, a precursor to the modern digital computer, was used to compile the 1890 U.S. Census. *(Photo courtesy of IBM Corporate Archives.)*

one-dimensional challenge that had already been addressed, but this was just the solution that directed them into the healthcare field.

"The whole opportunity came from billing systems," Patterson said during the company's 20th anniversary. "I've always thought that was ironic because ... we have spent 20 years being the company that understands clinical process and the mission [of this] industry."[35]

Medical Informatics—An Evolving Science

With MAWD as its first client, Patterson, Gorup, Illig & Associates (PGI) made a move into the hospital information systems field, part of a science known as medical informatics. One textbook defines the broad-ranging field of medical informatics as the science "that deals with the storage, retrieval, and optimal use of biomedical informa-

tion, data, and knowledge for problem-solving and decision-making."[36]

This segment of healthcare was launched in the United States in 1879—exactly 100 years before the formation of PGI—with Dr. John Shaw Billings' creation of a bibliography of medical articles called the Index Medicus.[37] Billings, a physician who was appointed director of the Army Surgeon General's Library after serving in field hospitals during the Civil War, set out to compile the first comprehensive index of medical journal articles from around the world.

The monthly index quickly evolved into the National Library of Medicine's multivolume resource that has been described as "America's greatest contribution to 19th century medicine."[38] In 1971, the index was transitioned into an electronic version called MEDLINE, which became a leading medical journal database.

While developing the collection that would eventually become the National Library of Medicine, Billings was asked to lend his problem-solving abilities to the U.S. Census Bureau. This invitation led to nothing less than the development of the first digital computer, which would bring medical informatics and every other industry into a new technological era.

Billings challenged a young engineer named Herman Hollerith to create a machine that could do the mechanical work of calculating population data and other statistics. Hollerith met the challenge with a punched-card data processing system designed to replace the "barbarous" system of manual counting used in previous decades.

Hollerith declared that "the records must be put in such shape that a machine could read them. This is most readily done by punching holes in cards or strips of paper, which perforations can then be used to control circuits through electromagnets operating counters or sorting mechanism, or both combined."[39]

Hollerith's Tabulating Machines successfully compiled the 1890 census ahead of schedule and under budget and launched a company that would later be named International Business Machines (IBM), maker of the first large-scale automatic digital computer.[40] Together, Billings and Hollerith melded medical expertise with engineering ingenuity to forge a new technological era. The forces that came together to launch *Cerner*'s first systems echoed this alliance of visionary thinking, and clinical and engineering know-how.

Computers in Medicine

The introduction of computers into medicine took place in the medical research field, and according to medical informatics pioneer Morris F. Collen, M.D., the 1960s and early 1970s were "golden years" for heavily funded research projects into computer technology. The funding came from three primary sources—the National Institutes of Health, the National Center for Health Services Research, and the Regional Medical Program.

"By the end of the '60s and early '70s," Collen wrote, "millions of dollars were being poured through these three streams, and computers began to spread all through the hospitals in this country."[41]

The outpouring slowed with the economic downturn of the mid-'70s, but by then the field had become established enough to produce the first international scientific meeting devoted solely to medical informatics. MEDINFO 1974, held in Stockholm, Sweden, featured 194 research papers, including six reports about the systems installed at El Camino Hospital in Mountain View, California.

The California-based Lockheed aerospace company was one of the first firms to apply its technological expertise to the development of a Hospital Information System (HIS). In 1966, the company began working with a group of physicians from the Mayo Clinic on an information system that they designed for the 464-bed community hospital in Mountain View.

In 1971, Lockheed sold that portion of its business to the Technicon Corp., a leader in computerized clinical laboratory systems. Technicon was ready to extend its successful lab automation into other hospital departments, and that year it created an automated system for the admissions office. This was followed by systems for lab test scheduling, I.V. ordering, pharmacy, and physician-entered medical orders.

The hospital laboratory, which handles massive amounts of data, as well as dramatic peaks in volume each day, was a logical place to begin introducing clinical information systems.

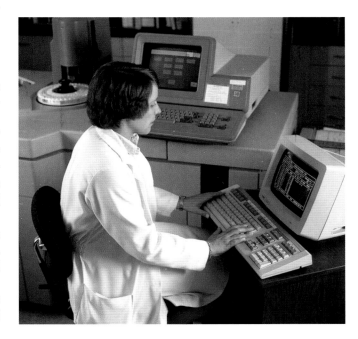

Computer terminals appeared throughout the hospital, and El Camino became the site of one of the first systems in which physicians could electronically enter orders—using a light pen that triggered a response on the computer screen—and view the results.

Doctors entered orders for lab work, medications, X-rays, and other procedures, which were then stored in the computer and sent to the appropriate departments. The El Camino system also included a Medical Information Library that allowed doctors to view medical information and articles on their computer screens. Although the system eliminated a lot of paper in the hospital, it did not replace the traditional paper medical chart; this early phase of automation was considered an order-entry and review tool only.

Technicon took its successful system to a handful of other hospitals in the 1970s, and by the time the three founders of *Cerner* began looking at healthcare IT in 1979, Technicon's systems were online in hospitals in San Francisco, California; Omaha, Nebraska; Fairfield, New Jersey; Portland, Maine; and the Clinical Center of the National Institutes of Health, in Bethesda, Maryland.[42]

Other facilities that implemented pioneering systems in the two decades before *Cerner* included the Medical Center at the University of Missouri-Columbia, which launched its system in 1964; the Texas Institute for Rehabilitation and Research at the Texas Medical Center at Houston, which grew out of a computer research system created during the 1950s; and the University of Vermont Medical Center in Burlington, which instituted its system in 1967.[43]

Preceding all of these was General Electric's Medinet project, an ambitious plan to build a comprehensive package of hospital information systems. But before GE had an opportunity to implement Medinet, the company dismantled the entire computer technology segment of its business. Later, GE would re-enter medical informatics as part of its Medical Systems business.

Other early pioneers who were legends in the history of medical informatics were Massachusetts General Hospital in Boston and the Kaiser Permanente company in Oakland, California.

Medical research brought computers into clinical laboratories in the early years of medical informatics. Radiology, electrocardiology, and pharmacy were among the first departments to embrace computer support, but the use of computers in hospitals during those years remained overwhelmingly administrative.

Gorup recalled the stark contrast between the minimal use of IT in healthcare and the explosive growth of its use in other industries in the late 1970s and early 1980s. "There were huge amounts of

---

By the mid-1970s, most hospitals were using computers to automate patient billing, collections, and third-party reimbursements. However, the paper medical chart, which could only be viewed by one person at a time, was still the norm. *(Photo by Antonia Felix.)*

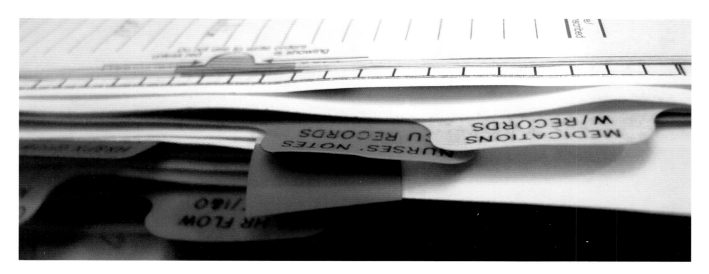

research, huge amounts of databases and a huge amount of information," he said, "and healthcare was just kind of moving along."[44]

Even though healthcare has made dramatic inroads since then, it still lags behind the advancements found in other types of businesses. "In an August 2004 meeting, one of our clients was talking about bar-coding for a patient's safety," Gorup said. "Twenty-five years ago, when Cliff and I were down at Cook, we did barcode scanners in the paint store. Healthcare adoption of technology, in many respects, from an information/operational flow is surprising. They adopt technology to improve some of the clinical evaluation processes, but in terms of the overall operation efficiency, how many decades has it been since bar-coding and scanning have been the accepted practice in Ma and Pa stores?"[45]

Slow to Change

By the mid-1970s, more than 85 percent of American hospitals were using computers for patient billing, collection, and third-party reimbursement services. This shift to computerized efficiency was similar to that occurring in other industries at the time, but hospitals were slow to invest in computerized clinical systems, patient records, and charts.

Why the reluctance to bring technology to the service of patient care? According to one study from the mid-1970s, four factors inhibited the forward pace of medical informatics at the patient-care level: poorly engineered computers, which were subject to breakdown and other problems, prevented good physician-computer interactions; computer programs simply duplicated physicians' tasks rather than adding to their capabilities; no proof yet existed that automated programs could positively affect patient care; and computer products did not easily transfer from one clinic or institution to another.[46]

At the very least, the evolving science of medical informatics had to resolve these problems before clinicians would embrace computers. To keep up with other industries that were already being advanced with the help of computer technology, medical informatics' greater challenge was to break new ground and lift healthcare to a new level of efficiency and performance.

By the time Patterson, Gorup, and Illig launched their business in 1979, lower-cost minicomputers that showed new promise for the advancement of medical informatics in clinical settings had been developed. Yet the vast majority of systems were separate programs specialized for specific departments that could not interface with one another. There were several reasons for developing these individual systems, as explained by G. Octo Barnett, M.D., a pioneer of medical informatics who developed the system at Massachusetts General Hospital:

The years of 1967–1972 were exciting times in the Laboratory.... The major organizing principle of our development was a "modular" approach. We argued that because of the difficulty in formulating a "total systems" plan, it was more productive to focus on identifying functional information processing units of medical activity and to provide well-defined and clearly bounded computer systems which could be explicitly integrated into the real and concrete medical needs of operating departments of the hospital. This modular approach ... sharply limited the initial start-up costs, and simplified the cost/benefit analysis since the computer program was closely linked to one specific operations unit.

An additional advantage which proved of great value was that this modular approach resulted in a "domino effect" where success in one department served as an attractive role model for development of modules for other departments. Lastly, a major advantage of the modular approach was that it facilitated flexibility and graceful evolution since we could make specific changes to one module without having a large, unforeseen or negative impact on other activities.[47]

As computer hardware became less expensive and processors got faster in the 1980s, the vision of integrated systems showed more promise. Hospitals and clinics began to use local area networks (LANs) to connect their systems, which allowed easier access to patient records by various caregivers throughout the hospital.

"The advent of network-linked microcomputers was probably the most significant development in the 1980s to advance clinical computing," Dr. Collen wrote.[48]

This was the exciting phase of advanced technology in which *Cerner* first outlined its vision for medical IT.

"The Status Quo Is Not Acceptable:" The Demand for Medical IT

When Patterson began working on MAWD's billing problem, the busy lab had an IT system that was typical of lab setups in the 1970s—a computer programmed to generate printed lab reports and bills. Although the software had been designed according to the pathologists' specifications, it was largely based on a well-known product called the Shared Hospital Accounting System (SHAS), a program developed by IBM in the 1960s.[49]

Using computers to replace handwritten reports and typed bills was a small step toward efficiency. But the fragmented, error-prone world of medicine was in desperate need of more sophisticated uses of technology.

The healthcare community was well aware of the factors that contributed to errors, and as *Cerner* grew along with a groundswell of demand for clinical technology, its associates became aware of the need for integrated systems that would improve safety.

But it was not until 1999 that the shortcomings of healthcare were put into terms that the general public could understand. That year, the Institute of Medicine (IOM), a think tank founded by the National Academy of Science, released a report titled *To Err Is Human: Building a Safer Health System*. Based on two old studies, the report concluded that medical errors cause the deaths of between 44,000 and 98,000 Americans each year.

"More people die in a given year as a result of medical errors than from motor vehicle accidents (43,458), breast cancer (42,297), or AIDS (16,516)," the report stated.[50]

Some common errors include the misidentification of patients and their needs (resulting in "wrong limb" amputations and other surgical mistakes); illegible physician handwriting, resulting in incorrect procedures and prescriptions; drug labeling mistakes (including the accidental dispensing of substances with similar names); and communication errors at all levels of care. Equally as startling, the studies showed that more than half of these deaths are preventable.

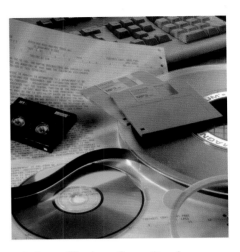

A 1999 report titled *To Err Is Human: Building a Safer Health System* by the National Academy of Science concluded that medical errors cause the deaths of 44,000 to 98,000 Americans each year. Many experts believe that information technology is the key to reducing medical mistakes.

In their summary of the effects of medical errors, the authors of *Internal Bleeding*, Drs. Wachter and Shojania, stated that the IOM report was not intended to point fingers at individual practitioners, but as a call to prioritize medical safety and efficiency.

"The real message, like ours, was that despite an unacceptably high rate of medical errors, most mistakes were the result of bad systems, not bad people," they wrote.[51]

In a television interview with Diane Sawyer on *Good Morning America*, which aired immediately after the report was released, Dr. Lucian Leape explained that inadequate systems are at the core of the problem. Leape, one of the authors of the studies on which the report was based, responded to Sawyer's comment that if the same rate of errors occurred in the airline industry, there would be a public outcry:

Well, you know, interestingly enough, airline pilots probably do have the same rate of errors as doctors and nurses in hospitals, but they have systems that keep those errors from causing planes to crash, and that's what this is all about. People in hospitals are careful, and they're not reckless, and we don't have a lot of negligent doctors, but they make mistakes, and what we have are systems that set them up to make mistakes and don't enable them to prevent those mistakes from causing injuries, and that's what the report is concerned about.[52]

Leape added that using computers to replace handwritten orders such as prescriptions can eliminate many errors.

"The computer doesn't forget," he said. "The computer doesn't let you write an order that's 10 times an overdose. Yes, you can make errors in programming, but those are really very rare compared to the kinds of mistakes we make every day when we write them by hand."[53]

Patterson elaborated upon the crucial role of technology in addressing the medical error epidemic in "The Mission of IT in Health Care," a chapter he contributed to a textbook called *Healthcare Information Management Systems*, published in 2004. He explained that the majority of IT systems continue to reinforce the status quo of fragmented, inefficient, shortsighted solutions. He maintained that the best alternative is to create smart, automated, unified systems that provide safeguards to reduce human error. That is precisely the type of solution that was formed as *Cerner* began designing its first clinical lab solution.

"The more promising answer is that IT is still the best hope for creating a new future for health care," Patterson wrote. "It is the implied answer in *To Err Is Human*."[54]

The writers of *To Err Is Human* proclaimed that hospitals have not been challenged by any incentives to create integrated, lifesaving systems that improve not only safety but quality of care. They described healthcare delivery as a "nonsystem" that is decentralized and dangerously fragmented and called for a new, proactive response.

"The status quo is not acceptable and cannot be tolerated any longer," the report stated. "Despite the cost pressures, liability constraints, resistance to change, and other seemingly insurmountable barriers, it is simply not acceptable for patients to be harmed by the same healthcare system that is supposed to offer healing and comfort."[55]

After more than a decade of working to create IT solutions at *Cerner*, Liane Lance personally experienced the potential for harm in medicine's "nonsystem" when she underwent treatment for breast cancer at age 37. Exactly as the studies and professional commentary have reported, she learned firsthand that the core problem is with the lack of a technologically unified system that puts the patient first. Although she said her caregivers were wonderful, the system in which they worked was not.

At every step of care she had to fill out forms about her medical history—for the internist, oncologist, general surgeon, plastic surgeon, lab, hospital pre-admissions, anesthesiologist, and others. This exhausting process forced her to focus on her diagnosis when she felt she should have been focusing on getting well. She said:

It's difficult to fill these forms out. It's difficult to write down the word "cancer" and see it on paper multiple times. This certainly adds to a patient's anxiety, and what I've learned is that even though the technology is available for this information to be in whatever format my clinicians need it to be for their particular specialty, I'm having to provide it. The burden is on me to provide it, as a patient, and what I feel strongly now is that I've done my job. I've done it many times, and the only job I should have left is to focus on getting well.... The patient's job is to get well. Not to shuttle forms, not to fill out forms, not to have to write down painful terms about themselves over and over again. Just to get well. That's all.[56]

Lance's experience highlighted one segment of the systemwide problem in healthcare delivery—patient records—that *Cerner* has sought to address. *Cerner*'s commitment to solve the "nonsystem" problem and eradicate painful, unnecessary experiences like Lance's began with the development of its first solution, *PathNet®*, in the early 1980s and has not wavered.

In 2002, long after *Cerner* had begun to address these issues, Patterson said, "I believe that healthcare is fundamentally broken. Across the country, the standard of care varies, even though the science is the same and even though the biology is the same. That does not have to be the case. We have the vision and the leadership inside this company to make a major difference in how healthcare works at the core level."[57]

Throughout the company's first decade, the mission was "to focus on clinical systems that maximized the efficient delivery of medical services—systems directly involved with the practice of medicine by clinicians throughout healthcare."[58]

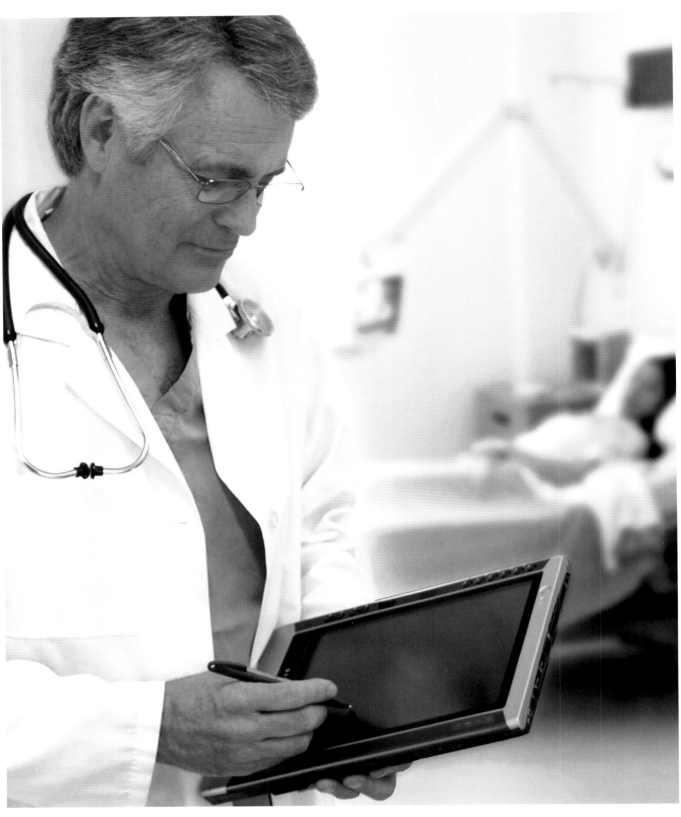

Technology assists physicians in updating patients' charts and accessing data from the latest medical research. *Cerner*'s goal is to create and enhance this technology for the benefit of patients.

CHAPTER TWO

THE ARCHITECTURE OF CHANGE

When we entered the marketplace, we targeted our offering to the sophisticated laboratory information system users, many of whom had already tried other lab systems before discovering PathNet®. We have been very successful with this marketplace because they appreciate the sophistication we have to offer. ... If I had to single out one concept which differentiates our offering and our approach from all others in the industry, I would focus on the fact that PathNet® is designed to be a total information system.

—Neal Patterson,
Cerner co-founder and CEO[1]

AS NEAL PATTERSON BECAME more entrenched in his work at the North Kansas City lab, he began to fully comprehend the critical need for information technology in medicine. While his two colleagues, Cliff Illig and Paul Gorup, worked with other clients in the Midwestern United States, Patterson began bringing together a team that would develop PGI's first clinical IT solution, *PathNet®*.

This solution for medical laboratories was based on PGI's *Health Network Architecture®*, an IT system designed with enough flexibility to grow and change along with the rapidly evolving healthcare industry. From its first application in two major hospitals, *PathNet®* stood out as a radically innovative laboratory solution. At the core of the system was a new type of software architecture that became a blueprint for the company's future clinical solutions and would address the specific needs of other sectors of healthcare.

A Vision for the Lab and Beyond

During its first year in business, PGI served several types of clients. Cliff Illig worked with transportation companies and manufacturers such as Brunson Instrument Company, a Kansas City-based maker of measuring tools, while Paul Gorup worked on systems for H&R Block and Cook Paint.

H&R Block quickly became one of the firm's most important clients when it chose PGI to automate some of its core business systems. The largest project PGI worked on was a cash-back/refund system, which allowed customers to get cash immediately when filing their tax returns through H&R Block.

These types of projects enabled PGI to finance Patterson's growing interest in medical IT software, and his success with MAWD's billing system helped him earn a solid reputation with the pathologists at the lab. When Dr. Terrance Dolan accepted a job as director of the laboratories at St. John Medical Center in Tulsa, Oklahoma, he once again turned to Patterson to help him fix a problem.

This time the challenge was broader, deeper, and much more complex. Dolan wanted to automate the various management tasks of the laboratories, and he believed Patterson could do it. Even though Patterson's solution at the Kansas City lab focused on billing, Dolan was convinced that Patterson had the skills and creativity to automate other elements of the laboratory.

This drawing from *Cerner*'s 1986 annual report illustrates the flexibility of the company's innovative *Health Network Architecture®*, which was designed to grow along with advancements in medicine and technology.

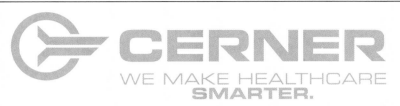

REFLECTS COMPANY'S VISION

IN 1984, PATTERSON, GORUP, ILLIG & Associates, Inc. (PGI) was getting ready to take its first solution, *PathNet*®, to the marketplace. The company hired a trio of advertising executives to help create a new company name that reflected technology and healthcare, and the advertising pros spent weeks brainstorming to come up with the perfect identity.

The ad executives were already working on sales brochures and other marketing materials, but nothing could be completed without the new company name.

"This is an era when the Intels and Microsofts were being named, too, and we were going for a tech name that had health in it," Patterson remembered.

With the clock ticking, suggestions such as Automated Information Management, Inc. (AIM) and Novus were rejected, and Patterson began to fear he would have to accept something he didn't really like. Then the ad executives produced a list of foreign words to look over, and one of them caught the eye of Jeanne Lillig, the seventh person to be employed by PGI, who went on to hold several executive roles within the company. She went to Patterson's office and told him there was one word from the list that stood out.

"What is it?" he asked her.

"*Cerner*," she said.

"That's it," Patterson said. "That's the name of the company."[1]

Cerner comes from the Latin word *cernere*, which means "to discern" or "to sift" with the senses or the mind. The Spanish definition is "to blossom," and the French word means "to encircle" or "encompass." These definitions reflected the expanding and integrative nature of the company's *Health Network Architecture*®, and PGI decided it fit perfectly.

And five years after PGI became *Cerner*, Lillig underwent a name change of her own when she and Patterson married.

Patterson noted that perhaps Dolan overestimated his abilities. "Terry thought that I probably knew a whole lot more about computers than I really did, but he had a lot of confidence in me and with the firm," he said.[2]

The task of automating several aspects of the labs at a large hospital was just the sort of challenge that inspired Patterson. Each lab department—hematology, chemistry, serology, urinalysis, microbiology, anatomical pathology, and blood bank—shared similar needs while demanding that attention be paid to their individual specialties. Each department's workload included dramatic peaks in volume each day and the ongoing need to quickly process large amounts of data.

In the spring of 1981, Dolan invited Patterson to present his initial ideas to the hospital's board of directors. Patterson said:

We had the opportunity to go down there and bid a contract, to develop from scratch a brand-new, state-of-the-art laboratory information system. I vividly remember [that] I had one sheet of paper where we had done a design of what we were going to build for Terry, and on this one sheet of paper was kind of the vision of the original PathNet® system. I was holding that picture up in the board meeting, pointing to it and basically saying, "Trust me. We will build this for you."[3]

They did trust him, and PGI won its first medical IT contract.

In the meantime, Patterson's growing familiarity with lab processes and healthcare in general was giving him new insights into the industry's IT needs. Perhaps in no other industry was quality information, provided in a timely manner, so essential.

During the early 1980s, healthcare providers were forced to choose from a handful of IT products. None of these systems addressed the management of clinical, operational, billing, and financial functions in a comprehensive way.

Patterson recognized an opportunity and envisioned IT solutions capable of solving the problems of the present and growing with the fast pace of high-tech innovation. As he and the rest of his software design team worked on *PathNet*®, they looked for similarities in the information needs of other clinical departments.

As *PathNet*® development advanced, the team realized that departments such as surgery, pharmacy, radiology, pulmonology, and critical care all shared with the laboratory many of the same needs for information. It quickly became evident that the ideal solution would be to develop a single information system that would ultimately bring the information from all clinical departments together, providing clinicians with a complete picture of each patient.

The team called this unified strategy, designed hand-in-hand with the development of *PathNet*®, *Health Network Architecture*® (HNA). The concept, a master blueprint for medical IT, was unique to the company and established a new model for the industry.

From this early stage in the company's history, HNA represented a commitment to unifying all clinical healthcare functions in an efficient and cost-effective way. HNA established a new standard for function, flexibility, organization, technology, system implementation, and client services. It became the framework around which the company would design every solution.[4]

From the start, PGI's strategy was to design solutions that could be easily modified or enhanced to take advantage of changes in computer hardware technology.

The HNA solution was designed to:

- Reduce the cost of developing additional comprehensive clinical information systems;
- Enable PGI to quickly adjust to technological developments in such areas as computer equipment, communications, and operating systems through the use of *InfraNet*, a proprietary software layered between the company's application products and manufacturer-provided technologies;
- Address the present and future needs of healthcare managers to identify, track, and price each event involved in the origination and processing of clinical information;
- Create common databases for clinical and management information to assure the

---

CERNER DOCTRINE

CULTURE

*C*ERNER'S COMMITMENT TO ITS solutions is deeply rooted in the spirit of the company. From the beginning, the company has recognized that it is the people at *Cerner* who envision the innovations, design and engineer the solutions, and serve the clients.

The company continuously attempts to foster a stimulating, fertile environment in which associates develop creative solutions. *Cerner*'s people share an attitude that prepares them to perform well and to care about the success of each client, and they are the driving force behind the company's growth.[1]

The *Cerner* culture has been developed by building and maintaining a positive, flexible work environment, where everyone has the chance to contribute. Associates respect one another's accomplishments and work hard to achieve success. When one team reaches a milestone, everyone celebrates because each individual is crucial to the company's success in the future.

unification of data necessary to improve patient care and reduce costs;

- Provide an open solution architecture that promoted ease of interface with financial/administrative functions, patient care, and other clinical systems;
- Address the needs of large and small clinical information system users by providing significant flexibility within all solution lines.[5]

As the company's quickly expanding solution line would reveal, HNA successfully delivered on all of these promises.

Incentives for Change

St. John Medical Center was eager to bring operational and fiscal order to its lab, which performed more procedural requests from physicians

than all other clinical departments combined. Like hospital administrators throughout the United States, those at St. John needed to bring a new level of efficiency to their facilities, especially the labor- and capital-intensive laboratory.

Tasks at the lab that needed a new level of attention included scheduling, controlling resources, tracking costs, and creating detailed cost analyses. These managerial concerns were becoming increasingly evident to healthcare providers throughout the nation when Patterson began thinking through a plan for St. John, and they culminated in government action in 1982, when Congress approved the Tax Equity and Fiscal Responsibility Act (TEFRA).

This law was an effort to control skyrocketing medical costs by changing the way physicians and institutions were reimbursed by Medicare. Through TEFRA, the federal government sought to force cost containment and greater efficiency in healthcare delivery.

Automation was inherent in TEFRA. Healthcare providers had no choice but to take active steps to streamline their services—including lab procedures—and technology was the only way to keep up with these complex demands. Along with the new law

---

Cerner developed its first solution, *PathNet®*, for the laboratory at St. John Medical Center in Tulsa, Oklahoma. *(Photo courtesy of St. John Medical Center.)*

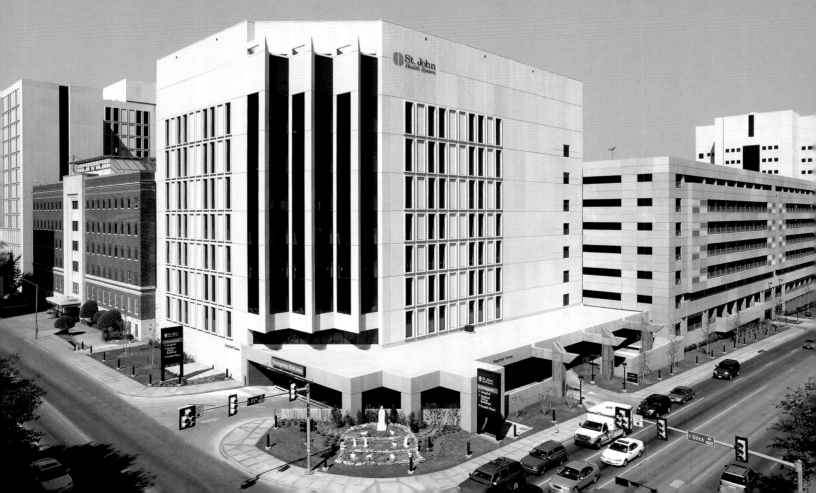

came a new set of acronyms: a prospective payment system (PPS) for acute care would be based on a set of diagnosis related groups (DRGs).

The key piece of information in this model was the patient's principal diagnosis, and the healthcare organization also coded and submitted additional information during the time the patient spent in the hospital. The DRG grouper—a computer software program that took the coded information and identified the patient's DRG category—considered the patient's age, gender, and discharge status. With all this information, a payment amount for the acute inpatient hospital visit would be set.

As Vice President and Chief Quality Officer Gay Johannes explained, this system was a major incentive for the medical industry to seek IT solutions. "TEFRA and the need to interface and leverage DRGs was a catalyst in moving healthcare providers from paper-based to electronic mediums to manage their business, and in doing so, providers had to respond by improving their operational efficiencies to maintain a steady cash flow of Medicare dollars."[6]

Liane Lance, *Cerner* vice president, related the effect of TEFRA on the company:

Cerner's primary focus in the early '80s was information systems for laboratories. TEFRA dramatically reduced profit margins for lab testing procedures and transformed labs from profit centers to cost centers. Cerner emerged as a change agent and partner to these physicians and institutions, offering solutions for labs to operate more efficiently, and spotted the critical value of the electronic medical record, automating systems across the continuum of care, and the need to connect it all.[7]

In addition to TEFRA, evolving medical technology demanded that healthcare facilities look for IT solutions. PGI soon realized that the answer lay in a unified system that could tie together information from different departments while automating operational tasks that address financial concerns. As the company's 1986 annual report asserted, *Cerner* had entered the medical IT business just when hospitals realized they had to learn how to manage the influx of computers and technology that were obviously there to stay. The report stated:

Through the Tax Equity and Fiscal Responsibility Act (TEFRA) of 1982, the U.S. government attempted to force cost containment and greater efficiency in healthcare delivery.

In the medical arena, computers are literally everywhere. They are being used to improve the precision, accuracy, timeliness, and cost of collecting patient data. The volumes of raw medical data produced by these devices, however, have greatly magnified the need for advanced clinical information systems to serve as "pipelines," "reservoirs," and "refineries" of information for physicians and medical professionals.

These factors have severely stressed the concept and form of traditional healthcare software. Further compounding this pressure has been the rapid deployment of newer mainframes and super minicomputers, causing the obsolescence of many computers on which traditional software systems

WORLD-CLASS QUALITY

IN JANUARY 2002, *CERNER* BECAME THE first U.S.-owned healthcare information technology company to earn ISO 9001:2000 certification.

Organizations that are awarded this coveted certification are acknowledged globally as industry leaders, committed to delivering quality products and services that are tested and proven to exceed customer expectations. Certification is evidence that all aspects of an organization's design, development, production, installation, and servicing meet quality and performance standards.

Established in 1947, the International Organization for Standardization (ISO), a worldwide federation of national standards bodies from some 140 countries, is currently the only true international standard embraced by the global marketplace because of its high standards for benchmark principles.

To become certified, *Cerner* elected to have all operational organizations, including software design and service delivery, audited by TUV Management Product Service, a globally recognized ISO registrar.

"As the lead auditor, I believe it is phenomenal and unprecedented that a company of *Cerner*'s size and complexity could achieve ISO 9001:2000 certification in only 10 months," said Larry Eaves, U.S. western region manager for TUV.[1]

Several of *Cerner*'s software solutions also fall into the category of medical devices required to be 510(K)-certified by the United States Food and Drug Administration (FDA) before release. These include the company's blood bank transfusion and donor devices, and radiologic imaging devices.

According to Shelley Looby, director of regulatory affairs at *Cerner*, the documentation process for 510(K) certification spans the entire lifecycle of the solution.

"It's an ongoing process," she said. "It actually starts when we are in the design phase of the device and continues until the device is no longer for sale."[2]

Although CEO Neal Patterson takes pride in the honor and others like it, he is quick to point out that certifications such as ISO 9001:2000 do not define quality; they are simply a byproduct of existing quality within an organization.

To achieve overall quality, Patterson often tells managers, an organization must embed pride in workmanship, define what constitutes "quality" from the client's point of view, assign responsibility to individuals to ensure standards are met, regularly evaluate quality using meaningful measurements, and continually pursue improvement of the current state.

were based.... In the face of this change we saw opportunity, and it was out of this environment that Cerner *emerged.*[8]

After conducting extensive research throughout 1980 and 1981, PGI concluded that there were no advanced medical IT systems on the market that embraced the dual needs of modern healthcare: delivering medical services to patients and controlling the costs of those services.

"Historically, healthcare information system companies had concentrated on providing systems that captured charges," explained the 1986 annual report. "Our plan was to focus on clinical systems that maximized the efficient delivery of medical services—systems directly involved with the practice of medicine by clinicians throughout healthcare."[9]

According to Patterson, the laboratory was the perfect place to begin transforming this vision into reality.

"The laboratory is the nexus of healthcare," he said. "A high percentage of things that go on in healthcare are connected to the laboratory. For the first half of the decade of the '80s, I was totally consumed by the laboratory, and in there was a huge opportunity to learn and listen and see."[10]

As a result, Patterson came to understand the relationship of the lab to the rest of the healthcare system, which was used to formulate the concept behind HNA. Patterson said:

There was a core process that made healthcare work, and it connected doctors and nurses and laboratories and radiology and ... pharmacy. It connected the person. So HNA was born out of half a decade of watching a major piece of health-care interact with the rest of healthcare, and it was [around] that set of relationships that we believed we could create an architecture.... I do believe that those three words—Health Network Architecture®—*capture a lot [of] what we saw back in the early '80s.*[11]

The *PathNet*® team worked around the clock to convert the solution at St. John, and without any precedents to follow, everyone learned on the job. "It's amazing what had to be done," Dolan recalled. "With software, no matter how well you design it and program it, there are always bugs, and of course, we had to fix the bugs on the fly." Patterson, Illig, and Gorup were with the team programming all day and fixing problems that came up. "In those early days, there was no really organized engineer-ing approach or quality control," Dolan said. "It was really by the seat of our pants so to speak, but that's how it was done. We were running a major regional center laboratory on this software, so we had to keep it going because it would adversely affect patient care if the software didn't keep running."[12]

From the beginning, the company had its eye on the future of healthcare IT and incorporated that vision into the development of the first lab solution. "The actual delivery of service, healthcare service, to the patient is a highly complex delivery system and requires very sophisticated systems," said Dolan. "One of the correct decisions we made when we developed *PathNet*® was that we intuitively felt the

data we were collecting would be very valuable in driving healthcare decisions in the future. So, as we came across data, the question was, do we keep it or not on electronic files? And we made the decision to keep everything we collected. Whether we knew what we were going to do with it or not, we felt we needed to collect it."[13]

Dolan added that this decision was vitally impor-tant to *Cerner*'s future development of an informa-tion database. "Seventy-seven percent of healthcare decisions are made on the results of a laboratory test," he explained. "Sixty percent of the healthcare database is made up of laboratory data, and one could extrapolate that 60 to 70 percent of total healthcare spending is delivered by the result of a lab test. We captured all those pieces of data from day one because intuitively we felt it would make sense, but it took us about 20 years to figure out how to use it. *Cerner*'s robust data set is now capitalizing on all that data we were capturing."[14]

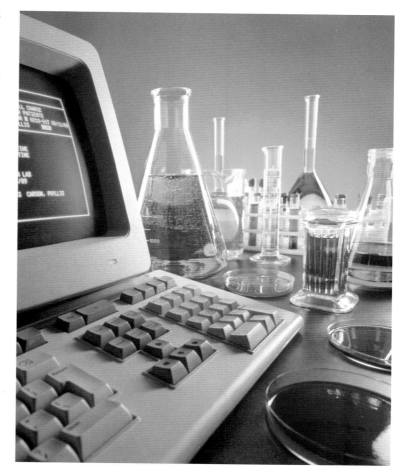

Neal Patterson described his company's *Health Network Architecture*® as a system that connected doctors, nurses, and departments such as the laboratory, radiology, and pharmacy. "It connected the person," Patterson said.

Trading Knowledge

Many of Patterson's ideas about healthcare IT grew out of months of meetings and conversations with James Flynn, M.D., the chief pathologist at Research Medical Center in Kansas City. This large, 508-bed hospital, situated on 60 acres, was in dire need of a data processing system that could support its clinical laboratory results.

The timing was perfect: Flynn needed an inventive computer systems company to automate his lab processes, and Patterson needed a medical expert to help him explore the complex needs of a lab system. According to Flynn, it was well-known around town that his hospital needed a new lab system, and this fact brought Patterson and Flynn together.

They began meeting after work, usually on Fridays, at the oyster bar at The Bristol, a long-time favorite hangout of Patterson, Illig, Gorup, and their associates. Flynn soon realized that Patterson's small but visionary company could offer the solutions Research Medical Center needed. Its challenges were much more complex than the budgetary concerns that had plagued the hospital, and it became Flynn's job to find a system that would meet its needs.

"Being the big hospital we were and not having the data processing support for laboratory result reporting, I was very anxious to get that support into the lab because the old pen-and-paper methods were just overwhelming us in volume," Flynn explained. "And there were certain errors that were associated with that, as well as delays, and getting the report to the consumer—the clinician—that I was anxious to interact with anyone who would have the prospect of creating a product that would help us out."[15]

Because PGI was a new company, its associates were eager to discuss an agreement.

"These fellows, being new into the area, were likely to provide that at a lower cost than more established vendors," Flynn said.[16]

At that time, Research Medical Center's method for disseminating lab information was a system of pneumatic tubes, in which handwritten reports were whisked from the lab to the nurse's station. "They were removed from the carrier and stuck into the chart," Flynn explained.[17]

This process created many opportunities for error, from poor handwriting to placement of the report in the wrong chart. As the physician responsible for finding a more efficient solution, Flynn was more than happy to brainstorm with Patterson about the specific needs of the lab.

"The laboratory, of course, is a place that creates a lot of numbers and a lot of information that goes from the lab to the bedside chart, and that is and was a very high-traffic area and therefore a good candidate for computer assistance," Flynn said.[18]

Patterson listened intently and quickly grasped the big picture, which gave Flynn a lot of confidence in his ability to develop an effective solution. Flynn said of Patterson:

> I gave him a lot of detail, and he could pull that together into what we now call a system to clarify how it was working for him as a systems person.... I happened to have been the ... frustrated laboratory director who was studying this business ... and [I was] also looking around the country ... at other vendors in the business of solving our problem.
>
> Actually, [PGI] didn't have a product at the time, but what impressed me with them, and especially with Neal, who was pretty much the head of this information gathering effort on their part, was that they ... listened very carefully to the people they were trying to create a product for, and they listened to their needs. I and others had visions of Neal coming into every meeting we had with a notepad and pencil, and he wrote constantly during those meetings.
>
> Those meetings included mostly him and perhaps another technical person on the PGI side, and my staff was a large group from which we picked senior technologists who actually knew at the bench level how this thing worked. He didn't squander the opportunity to get this right down to [every last] detail, which, of course, is where the code has to start.[19]

Flynn's in-depth knowledge of how the lab interacted with the rest of the hospital was central to Patterson's approach to developing *PathNet*®. Flynn also contributed vital insights into physicians' behavior and other elements of medicine that would be key to creating effective IT solutions. On those Friday nights, Flynn also talked to Patterson about technical problems and other challenges that had, thus far, hampered medical IT progress.

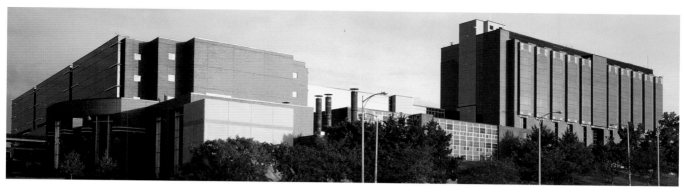

Flynn recalled the themes of many of those conversations:

> One thing I think I provided to Neal on those many Friday nights [when] we ... stood at the bar eating oysters and drinking martinis and beer ... was [information on] ... how doctors interact with each other. A fellow trained in finance really knows very little about the practice of medicine. We talked a lot about that, what motivated them, what they really cared about....
>
> We even got down to discussions of whether three-letter input into a keyboard was better than a mouse.... I'm a MacIntosh person, and of course, they were PC people, and there was a mix there among the technical issues of how do you get physicians to use these devices, which we're still dealing with.
>
> [We were even concerned with] the size of the font that a doctor would read in a patient's chart. I can recall back then when line printers were used, and it was difficult to change the size of a font.... When laser printers came along, which wasn't long after [PGI] got started, we had tremendous flexibility. Then the question was ... how much information can we put on a page, and how should it be organized? How do we create a page full of complex data for the consumption of the reader?[20]

Although Flynn discussed a lab system with Patterson from the earliest days of *PathNet®* development, his hospital was slow in deciding to actually purchase a new solution. Flynn had led an exhaustive comparative search for a company to meet Research Medical Center's needs and ultimately recommended PGI to his hospital administration, but three other hospitals went forward with a developmental/purchase agreement for *PathNet®* ahead of his facility.

In 1983, *Cerner* implemented *Pathnet®* at North Kansas City Hospital, whose early healthcare facilities are depicted in this vintage photo. The 451-bed hospital is located across from present-day *Cerner* World Headquarters. *(Photo courtesy of North Kansas City Hospital.)*

"When we made that recommendation, it took them a long time to make the decision to allocate that kind of capital to our problem," Flynn said. "That hospital, like hospitals in general, [has] many places to put [its] money, and they delayed a long time. So ours was the fourth installation, but following that installation it was, at least for me, for us, a dramatic change from the shingled, handwritten paper reports that went by way of pneumatic tube to the nurses' station."[21]

Patterson also discussed his ideas with Jim Mongan, M.D., then-executive director of Truman Medical Center in Kansas City, who shared an interest in automating many aspects of care delivery. Mongan, currently president and CEO of Partners Health Care, told Patterson, "We are all using managed care as a noun, and nobody is actually managing care or using it as a verb."[22]

Mongan was serving on ProPAC, the advisory commission set up by the Congress to make recommendations about Medicare reimbursement to hospitals, when he had these discussions with Patterson. "I was very interested in health policy and health payment issues, and Neal certainly had those strong interests also. We began to see each other as people who had a broad vision of where this health system might go if it were properly linked with electronic records that could be used to enhance the efficiency of care."[23]

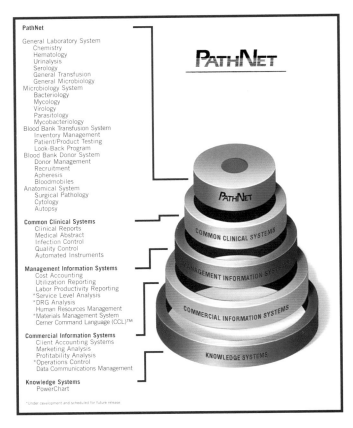

Above: The *PathNet*® cylinder model illustrates the multilayered, integrative design of the solution and the *Health Network Architecture*® on which it is based.

Right: Neal Patterson uses the cylinder model in 1986 to explain *PathNet*®'s capabilities.

The Cylinder Model

The PGI team that developed *PathNet*® included medical technicians from the four medical centers in which the first *PathNet*® solutions were implemented. These technicians included Nancy Moore from St. John Medical Center in Tulsa, Vanetta Wick and Liane Lance from North Kansas City Hospital, and Janice Woods from Research Medical Center. Woods recalled the day that Patterson arrived for a meeting to talk to Flynn and other technicians about his vision of a lab solution for their hospital. He was armed with a visual aid to help describe his ideas that is now legendary in *Cerner* circles. She said:

They basically came with an 8.5-by-11 piece of paper that had boxes on it that described the laboratory modules that they saw needed to be developed. Of course, at that time, there ... was practically nothing developed, but they basically had this clear picture in their minds of what the lab information system should look like, and the interesting thing about that was that virtually every one of those boxes came to fruition before it was all over. So they had a very clear idea very early on of exactly what they decided that they needed to do.[24]

The boxes in the illustration would soon become segments in a cylindrical model that *Cerner* would develop over the years.

The founders were heavily involved in *PathNet*® design at every level. Illig focused on the technical design and architecture, while Patterson concentrated on the solution's functionality, determining how it would help the lab. Gorup drove the development process as *PathNet*® moved toward its first installation in a hospital lab.[25]

The technicians who were hired to help Patterson and Illig develop the system had a clear-cut role during that time, which, according to Woods, was to "help them figure out what a laboratory information system needed to do." She added that technicians were better suited than pathologists for this task, as they used the system and were familiar with the territory. "Pathologists sort of have the big, grand scheme in mind," she said, which does

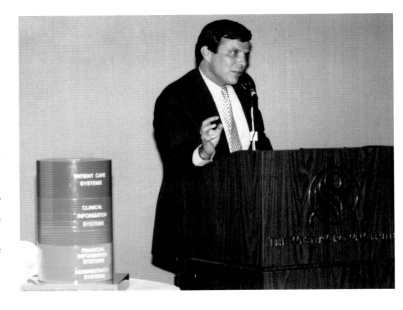

not lend itself easily to minute details of writing computer code.[26]

The development of *PathNet*®—purely a process of trial and error—required close working relationships between the PGI team and the medical personnel. "Basically," Woods explained, "you had to put a piece of code out there, try it, see if it worked, see if it was what the end users liked and what they could use, come back, give them feedback, and then make changes."[27]

Patterson's team was unique, in that it always kept in mind the crucial need for both clinical and management functions in its lab solution, which would enable caregivers to meet the new TEFRA requirements. Before *PathNet*® was developed, most lab systems had been designed to manage billing alone and lacked the ability to address cost analysis, as well as additional business concerns. A few other systems were designed to meet the needs of a single physician.

"Most of the healthcare systems at that time had as their genesis a doc, a pathologist who had an idea and got some programmers ... and went off and developed a system to satisfy the scientific needs of the laboratory," said Rick Fiske, the company's vice president of operations at the time. "But the people that were the genesis of it didn't have any kind of real structured business background."[28]

PGI, on the other hand, brought an additional set of skills to the task.

"These guys came into it from a whole different perspective," Fiske said. "They came into it to design, solve a business problem, and identified ways to do it that were just different than the rest of the world and much deeper in scope. They relied on their clients for technical knowledge, and they provided the systems knowledge and the design and ended up with a very unique design in the business."[29]

The end result of years of development work was the implementation of *PathNet*® at St. John Medical Center in Tulsa in August 1982; at North Kansas City Hospital in May 1983; at St. John's Hospital in Leavenworth, Kansas, in August 1983; and at Research Medical Center in Kansas City in October of that year.

Patterson recalled the round-the-clock work during the St. John conversion in Tulsa, where the team rented one room at the Residence Inn and slept in shifts.

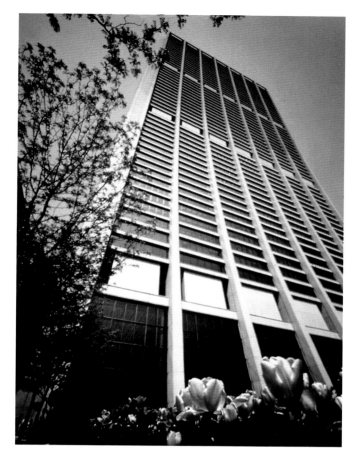

In 1983, *Cerner* received its first venture capital deal—for $1.5 million—from First Chicago Capital Corporation, which was housed in a downtown Chicago skyscraper, now called Chase Tower. *(Photo courtesy of Chase and BankOne.)*

"It was really wonderful," he said. "We had a kitchen there. We just thought that was the ... neat[est] thing versus motel rooms."[30] But with someone always in the room, there wasn't much of an opportunity for privacy and rest outside of the "shift schedule." Patterson solved this problem by finding a quiet corner of the hospital in a most unlikely place.

"I found if I'd go to the morgue that people would look for me every other place except there. I'd go in and get a little bit of sleep." Sometimes he slept on a cot, but at other times he climbed on top of one of the metal tables where, perhaps only a short time before, a corpse had been laid out. "It was always cold, [and] you were always a little bit on alert if you heard something," he said.[31]

Funding the Vision

By 1982, it had become clear to PGI that the company would not be able to finish developing *PathNet®* without a new source of cash, and that year Patterson began the daunting task of funding his vision.

"I had added to my list to go out and find some money and raise some capital, probably never even having heard of the term venture capital at that stage," he recalled. "I was quite naïve."[32]

The first year he tried raising money in Kansas City, where the company had already exhausted all of its sources for bank loans.

"I talked to everybody in town that we could think of that would be a potential investor," Patterson said. "When I'm speaking publicly in Kansas City, one of my lines that I use from time to time is that the reason most people know me personally here in Kansas City is that at one point in time or the other, I tried to borrow money from them. It was a very frustrating year."[33]

Patterson and his colleagues knew that they could build a company around *PathNet®* and their innovative software architecture, but after a year of looking for funding close to home, they were no closer to financing it. Patterson was getting discouraged, but he found new hope in a bright, energetic new associate named Hal Oppenheimer. A graduate of Harvard Business School, Oppenheimer shared Patterson's proactive and enthusiastic outlook.

The company hired Oppenheimer to help raise money, and he helped develop a plan to arrange a private equity placement in which funds came from individuals. Patterson was not in love with the idea, however. "It was a very ugly way of raising money," he remarked.[34]

In November 1983, he and Oppenheimer attended an *INC* magazine seminar, "How to Raise Venture Capital," in Chicago in hopes of finding a better way. The decision was an excellent one due to some good old-fashioned networking. At the seminar, Oppenheimer looked up a fellow Harvard MBA graduate, Paul Finnegan, who was working for First Chicago Capital Corporation and immediately got a dinner invitation.

"I'd have dinner, breakfast, lunch with anybody if there is a chance of raising money," Patterson recalled.[35]

Finnegan was the first venture capitalist Patterson had spoken to, and during dinner Patterson described all the great things his young company was doing—its visionary architecture and innovative *PathNet®* developments.

The next day, while seated in a large auditorium with approximately 1,000 other seminar attendees, Patterson looked across the room and spotted Finnegan scanning the crowd. Patterson knew Finnegan was looking for him and Oppenheimer.

"My blood pressure shot up," Patterson said. "My adrenaline was pumping. I knew we had him on the hook."[36]

Finnegan found them in the crowd and asked if there was any chance they could come by the First Chicago Capital offices before they left town. Patterson, not wanting to appear desperate, said, "Sure. It will be a little tough, but sure, we'll make it."[37]

Patterson and Oppenheimer attended the meeting, and in two weeks they managed to close a deal for $1.5 million. What Patterson had failed to do in Kansas City in nearly a year and a half, he had accomplished in just two weeks in Chicago. For the young company, that was cause for jubilation.

"We thought we had all the answers in the world," Patterson said. "We were going to go attack the world."[38]

***PathNet®*
Laboratory Solutions**

Designed on a Texas Instruments platform, *PathNet®* successfully met the demanding needs of the laboratory by performing the following functions:

- Processing and scheduling test requests from physicians and tracking the flow of events within the laboratory departments;
- Collecting and validating test results and their interpretations;
- Organizing the data from all procedures for optimum presentation to the physician;
- Providing for quality control and quality assurance over the entire process;
- Maintaining clinical information for short-term and long-term storage and retrieval;
- Measuring costs, employee productivity, and resource utilization for management;

• Communicating clinical information to patient care areas and to the healthcare provider's other data processing facilities.[39]

PathNet®'s ability to track several activities answered the need for software that could manage the lab's complex procedures. This unique design made *PathNet*® stand out from the competition in that it defined and tracked each specific activity, event, or procedure; specified exactly who performed or failed to perform an event; and specified when and where each event took place. This level of detail gave healthcare managers a great deal of control over daily operations.

The earliest *PathNet*® Laboratory Information System solutions were grouped into five broad categories that addressed different sets of client needs and could be converted alone or in combination, as necessary. The General Laboratory solution, released in 1982, automates the information flow of the chemistry, hematology, urinalysis, serology, toxicology, coagulation, immunology, general transfusion, and general microbiology sections of the general laboratory. Once collected, specimens are automatically loaded in priority sequence to the appropriate workstation for testing and result recording. The system validates results and quickly alerts the technologist to critical situations and entry errors.

The Microbiology solution, released in 1983, automates the information flow of the bacteriology, mycology, virology, parasitology, and mycobacteriology sections of the microbiology lab. The system tracks and reports testing directed at identifying and stopping the growth of bacteriological pathogenic organisms present in both humans and animals. Online worksheets allow the technologists to record observations and results, eliminating much of the documentation required in a conventional manual system.

The Blood Bank Transfusion solution, released in 1985, automates the inventory and transfusion requirements of the blood bank. The system includes

The microbiology lab at Methodist Hospital in Houston converted to *PathNet*® in 1987. Online worksheets allow technologists to record observations and results, eliminating a great deal of manual documentation.

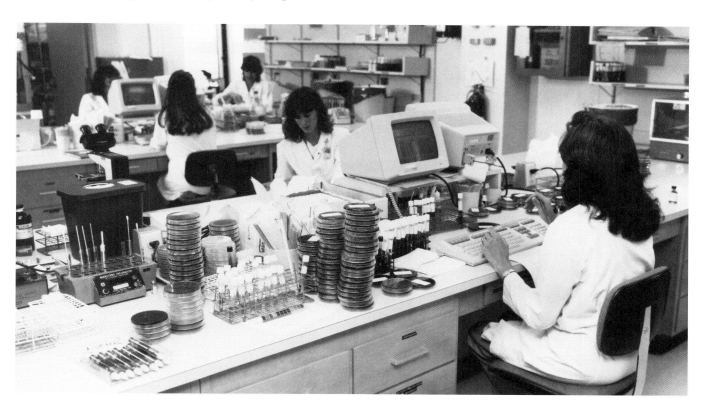

bar code labels and readers that provide efficiency and help ensure accuracy. A related system, the Blood Bank Donor solution, released in 1986, provides donor scheduling and long-term donor and transfusion record-keeping. Designed to properly match service requirements with available donors, this system was fully unified with the Blood Bank Transfusion solution and created for use in a hospital or community blood bank.

The fifth category, Anatomic Pathology, automates the information flow of the surgical pathology, cytology, autopsy, and histology sections of the pathology lab. The system advances the procedural flow of pathology specimens through the lab and automatically notifies the pathologist of prior procedures and diagnoses for the patient. A text editor simplifies the entry of reports, including the automatic coding of reported diagnoses to enable archival storage and access.[40]

Janice Woods described *PathNet*® as a "virtually hands-off" system, unlike four other lab information systems with which she is familiar.

"If you have an instrument that is able to read a barcode," she explained, "all you need to do is label the tube with a barcode, put the tube on the instrument, and with a combination of a bidirectional interface and a feature that they call auto-verification, the results could be printing on the nursing units virtually without any interaction. You label the tube, put it on the instrument, and the next thing you know, the results are printing on the floor."[41]

PathNet® allows lab technicians to label specimens with a barcode, scan the barcode, and ultimately make the results available to nursing units more quickly.

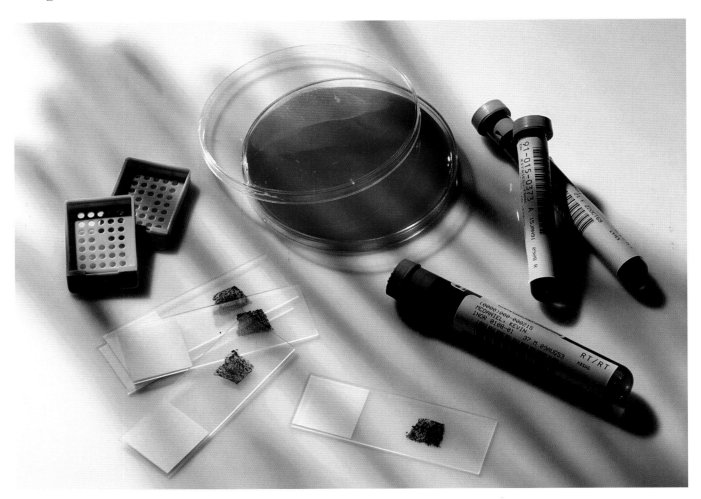

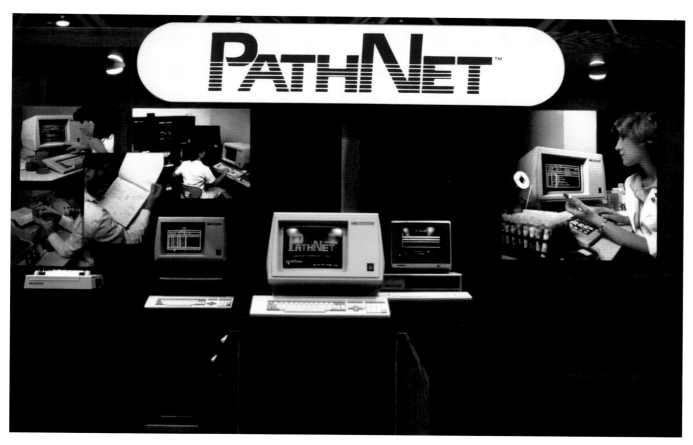

PathNet®'s speed and efficiency quickly caught on as the new standard of information exchange between the lab and other medical departments at Woods' hospital. When a severe electrical storm caused some hardware problems at Research Medical Center, the doctors learned just how thoroughly they had come to depend upon *PathNet*®'s high pace and efficiency.

"I remember our medical director at the time being called to a meeting at the Department of Surgery because they were concerned," Woods said. "Our computer system had gone down because of the storm. This had nothing to do with *PathNet*®, but the surgeons were irate because they were so used to getting the information in such a timely way—basically before they even started their surgeries at seven o'clock in the morning—that they were just beside themselves this one particular day when things went bad."[42]

The doctors asked the medical director what they should expect the next time a storm knocked out hardware. He told them they should just remember what it was like before they had a computer system. "I thought that just said it all," Woods said.[43]

This trade show booth helped *Cerner* introduce *PathNet*® to the commercial marketplace in the spring of 1984. In just two years, the company had finalized agreements with 41 clients to implement the solution at 49 facilities.

PathNet® Hits the Market

After working through most of the challenges at the first four *PathNet*® implementation facilities, the solution was brought to the commercial market in the spring of 1984. Two years later, the company had made agreements with 41 clients to implement the solution at 49 facilities. This fast pace of growth did not go unnoticed in the medical IT industry and in 1986 prompted the trade magazine *Healthcare Computing & Communications* to take a closer look at the small upstart company with an article titled, "Who Are Those Guys at *Cerner* Corporation?"

The article announced that *Cerner*'s gross revenues had increased 500 percent between 1984 and 1985, with staff growth of 400 percent.

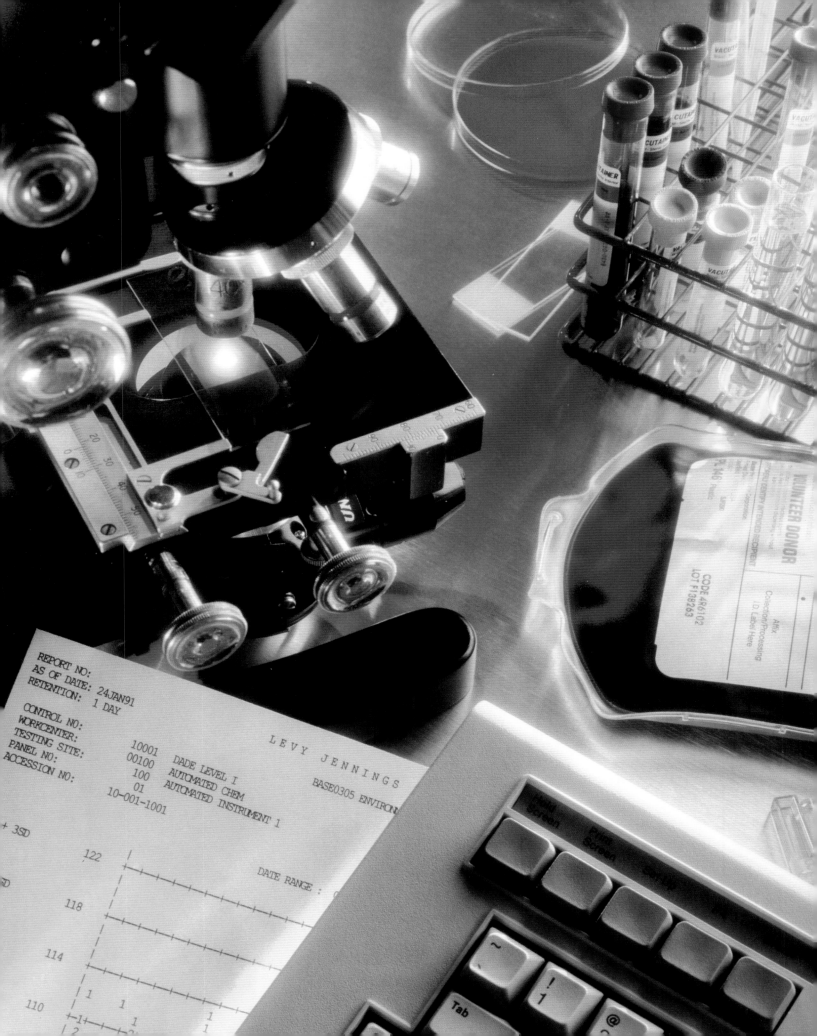

LEVY JENNINGS

REPORT NO:
AS OF DATE: 24JAN91
RETENTION: 1 DAY

CONTROL NO:
WORKCENTER:
TESTING SITE: 10001   DADE LEVEL I
PANEL NO: 00100   AUTOMATED CHEM   BASE0305 ENVIRON
ACCESSION NO: 100   AUTOMATED INSTRUMENT 1
                     01
                     10-001-1001

+ 3SD

        122

        118

        114

        110

Opposite: Over the years, the *PathNet®* line expanded to include the Human Leukocyte Antigen (HLA) solution that supports organ transplant programs and Specimen Management, which automates the collection, processing, and storage of specimens for laboratory testing.

"They continue to lure some of the brightest talent in the industry because of their long-term, yet innovative approach to the market and the *PathNet®* product," the magazine reported. *Cerner's* high profile in the industry was evident, as "in the last two years *Cerner* has left knowledgeable industry professionals and competitors on the edge of their chairs as three of the four largest hospital management corporations in the country have selected *PathNet®* over all other laboratory systems available."[44]

The article quoted Terry Armstrong, assistant vice president of Hospital Corporation of America (HCA), on his facility's reason for choosing *Cerner*: "We looked at all the laboratory systems on the market and found *PathNet®* the most functional. We feel good about *Cerner's* recent successes because we chose them three years ago, long before anyone else saw their product genius. Since that time we have experienced an excellent working relationship with *Cerner*."[45]

The article's author, Loran Walker, continued:

Many industry observers ... are wondering how Cerner has risen to the top so quickly, and if they can indeed keep up such a charmed life. Neal Patterson, president and chief executive officer of Cerner, said, "Let them wait. We've only begun to stimulate this market. We're going to force the competition to question whether or not they know how to manage a software product for any length of time, to question whether or not they know how to manage technology for more than seven years. We're going to challenge their concepts of product management by example."[46]

The article concluded with a reference to a scene from the film *Butch Cassidy and the Sundance Kid*, when Cassidy asked Sundance, "Who are those guys?" as they fled from a posse. Walker wrote, "Today that question is being asked by pathologists,

lab managers, and hospital administrators alike. And the answer is rapidly unfolding as *Cerner's* rising star reaches the top of the ... industry."[47]

By 2004, the five original *PathNet®* solutions had been further developed, and the line expanded to include two new solutions. The Human Leukocyte Antigen (HLA) solution supports organ transplant programs by automating clinical, financial, and managerial processes associated with HLA typing, antibody screening, crossmatching, and recipient-donor matching. The HLA solution addresses all processes including specimen setup, testing result entry, and review functions. The system also provides management and statistical report options to provide information necessary for the optimal operation of the HLA laboratory.

The second new laboratory solution, Specimen Management, automates the activities surrounding the collection, processing, and storage of specimens for laboratory testing. Like all *PathNet®* solutions, it was designed to streamline processes, improve turnaround times and efficiency, reduce costs, and improve specimen quality. This solution handles the scheduling of future orders, printing collection lists and labels, logging specimens into the lab, tracking specimen containers as they are transported between locations within and between laboratories, and other components of specimen handling in the lab.

Cerner's 1988 annual report described the strategy of *PathNet®* and the *Health Network Architecture®* upon which it is based as part of an expanding network of systems that "can control the most data in the most usable form, greatly affecting the quality of care the patient receives."[48] *PathNet®* set the stage for all future *Cerner* solutions, which continue to meet the challenges that have been facing the medical industry for decades.

"It is necessary that we manage personnel, equipment and processes, both within the departments and throughout the institution," the report stated. "It is imperative, once the results are ready, that we present the clinical information comprehensively and that we emphasize the clinically significant attributes of the data, thereby increasing its value to the clinical decision-makers. This is what we do."[49]

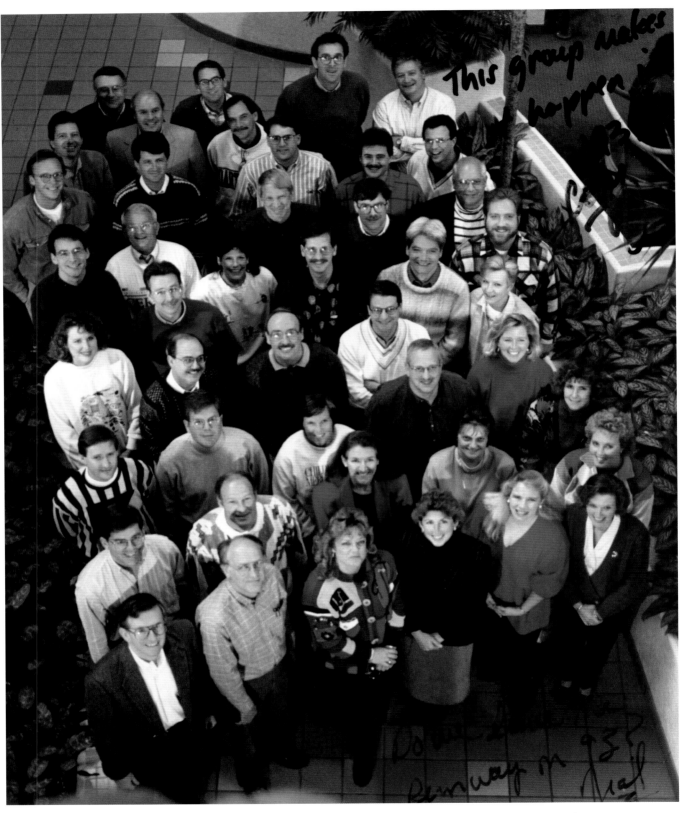

A group of *Cerner* associates gathers at a company meeting in 1993. Over the years, the company's founders worked hard to develop a workplace culture at *Cerner* that would help attract and retain the top talent in the industry.

CHAPTER THREE

CREATING A SYSTEM–AND A COMPANY–THAT CARES

Everything we do is for the betterment of human life.

—Liane Lance, *Cerner* vice president[1]

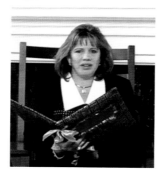

THROUGHOUT ITS HISTORY, *Cerner* has demonstrated innovation in work style, as well as in the development of groundbreaking healthcare solutions. As new clinical systems were developed, the company's founders became even more committed to creating and maintaining a unique culture at *Cerner* that reflected their vision of the ideal work environment.

At the heart of this culture are philosophical tenets that the founders learned from legendary Kansas City businessman and philanthropist Ewing Marion Kauffman, founder of the pharmaceutical giant Marion Laboratories. Patterson and Illig credit Kauffman with helping them develop a workplace that continues to attract the high level of talent that has made *Cerner* into a global leader in medical information technology.

Total Commitment: "A Christmas Story"

From the beginning, *Cerner* sought out individuals who were highly motivated and deeply committed to the company's vision. When *Cerner* introduced *PathNet*® to the marketplace in 1984, the development team was designing an updated version of the solution for Community Hospital East of Indianapolis, a 550-bed hospital and part of a four-hospital system in the city. Still a small company, *Cerner* put every resource it had into making

version 2.2 of *PathNet*® work at the busy hospital. As the holiday season drew near, however, the challenges of the conversion seemed to be endless.

The commitment of *Cerner* associates to work through the problems at this hectic time of year reflected the attitude that pervaded the company during its formative years and continue to define it 25 years later. This dedication is illustrated in the story of the Indianapolis conversion, which Liane Lance related in a company video titled "A Christmas Story." The following is Lance's narrative:

I want to tell you about a very special Christmas. Back in 1984, there were only 55 associates in the company. We were not yet a publicly traded company, and money was tight. In 1983, we had started a large rewrite of the PathNet® *software, which was the only product that we had at the time. The site where we were piloting this was the Community Hospitals of Indianapolis (CHI). The CHI implementation was a very important one to us because we were replacing what was, at the time,*

Liane Lance relates "A Christmas Story" about associates' dedication during the holiday season conversion of *PathNet*® at Community Hospitals of Indianapolis.

our largest competitor in the laboratory marketplace. Everyone was watching.[2]

Only two days into the conversion, the associates realized that the project was going to be a significant challenge. Exhausted and under an increasing amount of pressure, they persevered working round the clock. Lance continued:

By December 12, there were now 55 or 54 associates up in Indianapolis. We only left one person back in Kansas City to answer the phones. One med-tech in the lab was so frustrated and so angry that when Neal went in one day and asked, "How's it going?" she picked up a chair and threw it at him.

By December 22, we had to make a decision about keeping the system running over the holidays. Neal gathered all the Cerner *associates in the library and closed the doors. He said that it was our decision to make about whether or not we would turn the system off. We had two choices: a) turn it off and help them revert back to their MedLab system with the hope that they'd give us another chance; or b) keep the system running and try and fix the things that weren't working. Then he walked out of the room, outside, into the dark where it was snowing.*

When he came back in, the decision had been made to leave the system running and fight our way through.[3]

Patterson, Lance, and Randy Block remained at the site to ensure that the system stayed up, while the rest of the associates made a brief trip home. What could have been a disheartening holiday turned upbeat when Liane's husband Steven, arrived, setting up a surprise Christmas tree and preparing a special meal for the tired team. For dessert, they visited the home of the lab manager where Steven entertained them with piano music and Christmas carols. While their hearts were back home with family and friends, Lance recalled, "I will never forget standing there and knowing that it was the right thing for me to be doing."[4]

Several days later, the rest of the *Cerner* team returned, and the site was rapidly turned around. According to Lance, the product became incredibly successful. "It was one of the most enduring mem-

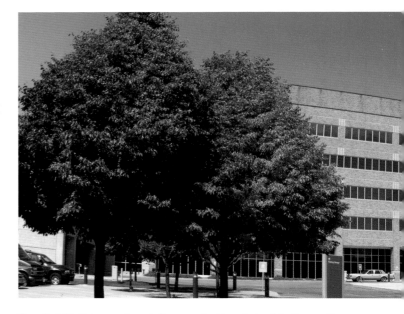

The *PathNet*® conversion at Community Hospitals of Indianapolis, part of Community Health Network, was critical to *Cerner*'s future success since the young company replaced the system developed by its main competitor. *(Photo courtesy of Community Health Network.)*

ories of my career. And as it turns out, it was the best Christmas that I ever had," she said.[5]

Bryan Ince, one of the software developers who worked on the Indianapolis conversion, shared another example of the commitment that *Cerner* associates showed during this early client experience. Ince, now vice president of development for *Cerner* Knowledge and Discovery, was troubled by a situation that occurred just outside the IT area in which he and the rest of the team were working. He recalled:

The data center was next to the outpatient clinic. On the morning of conversion I walked out the door of the data center, and I saw a line of people spilling out of the clinic area and into the hallway. There were young kids fidgeting around and elderly people standing, leaning, sitting on the floor. It was December, so everyone had heavy winter coats, which were laying around everywhere. I asked someone who worked there if this was normal; she glared at me and said 'No, it's the new computer system.'

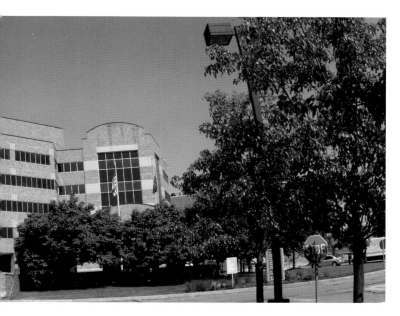

I made my way to the front of the line to see what was going on. I saw that the problem was that the phlebotomist was standing by the label printer waiting for lab specimen labels to come out. They were trickling out at a very slow rate, and that was causing the backlog of people. That was the part of the system that I had been working on. I was stunned. It was my fault that all of these people were stuck in line for so long.

That night, and the next night, I redesigned and rewrote our entire approach to how we printed lab specimen labels. I didn't leave until it was fixed because I couldn't walk past that line of people to go back to the hotel and get sleep. It wasn't just me; there were a bunch of us in that room going around the clock. I remember Rich Famuliner, Phil Fulks, Paul Gorup, Neal Patterson, Liane Lance, Stan Wollard, and probably others who never left the data center during that critical time.[6]

The Kauffman Legacy

The dedication of *Cerner* associates is part of a company culture that has been inspired by several factors, one of which was the philosophy of an almost larger-than-life figure from the Kansas City business community. Patterson and Illig found a world-class business mentor in entrepreneur and philanthropist Ewing Marion Kauffman (1916–1993), the most famous son of Kansas City

and the one who had left perhaps the biggest mark on the community.

Their brief encounters with Kauffman, affectionately known as "Mr. K" made a lasting impression, and the lessons they learned from his well-documented life inspired their beliefs about workplace culture.

Kauffman spent his early childhood on a farm in Missouri, where, like Patterson, he witnessed firsthand the risks involved in that way of life. Three years of flooding and ruined crops forced the family to quit farming and move to Kansas City. After serving in the Navy during World War II, Kauffman worked as a pharmaceutical salesman and, in 1950, launched his own drug company, Marion Laboratories, Inc.

Working out of the basement of his home, Kauffman concentrated on selling tablets and injectible medications that doctors had begun using regularly in the 1950s as an alternative to prescribing pills. Kauffman used his middle name for his company so customers wouldn't know it was a one-man operation.[7]

Marion quickly became a booming enterprise that joined the ranks of the world's major pharmaceutical companies. When the company was sold to Merrell Dow in 1989, it was an international,

---

CERNER DOCTRINE

KNOWLEDGE ORGANIZATION

IN A SUCCESSFUL COMPANY, KNOWledge is valued and nurtured as the greatest asset of the organization. Learning is a lifelong process for companies and individuals; and continuous learning, ongoing improvement, and evolution drive a healthy company.

Risk-taking and learning from mistakes also make up the dynamic process that runs the knowledge organization.

diversified pharmaceutical giant with annual sales of nearly $1 billion.[8]

Kauffman believed deeply in giving back to the community, and in addition to providing thousands of jobs through his company, he enhanced the economy of Kansas City in several ways. One of his most famous ventures was bringing major league baseball to town by establishing the Kansas City Royals in 1968. Royals Stadium was re-named Kauffman Stadium in his honor a few months before he died in 1993.

During the mid–1960s, Kauffman also used his wealth to establish a foundation that has become a significant source of funding for innovations that advance entrepreneurship and education. The Kauffman Foundation strives to foster an environment nationwide in which entrepreneurs at all levels can succeed. The Foundation focuses its educational programming on raising the academic achievement of children in Kansas City, placing a special emphasis on building their mathematics and science skills.[9]

As young entrepreneurs in the Kansas City business community, Patterson and Illig were well aware of Kauffman, his enormous success, and the business philosophy that stood behind it all. They had met him at various functions, as well as through a few memorable meetings at which Kauffman offered advice about their young company. Patterson missed one opportunity, however, to spend an entire afternoon with Kauffman, a decision he called "one of my regrets in life."[10]

Patterson had been invited to lunch at the Kansas City Club, where Kauffman happened to play cards regularly. Patterson arrived early and was sitting on a couch, when Kauffman walked by, recognized Patterson, and stopped to chat. Kauffman mentioned that he and his friends were short a player that day.

"Here's this legend," Patterson recalled, "and he said, 'Do you want to play gin?' I froze. I went through all the things I had to do that afternoon." Patterson declined the invitation, convinced that his obligations that day were too important to postpone. "I'm sure it would have changed my life to play cards with him," Patterson said. As a young person launching a new business, Patterson said, "you're in the most learnable part of your life. If [a leader has] a map, you want to copy it. Mr. K was very good at the

principles of things to do. As an entrepreneur, you seek people who have survived."[11]

Kauffman's fundamental philosophy was, "Treat others as you want to be treated." More than a scripture-inspired golden rule, Kauffman considered this guideline to be the key to success in all areas of life. This tenet, he stated, "is the happiest principle by which to live and the most intelligent principle by which to do business and make money!"[12]

The second and third of Kauffman's three main philosophies, according to biographer Anne Morgan, were, "Those that produce should share the rewards," and "Give back to the community."[13] Each of these ideas made a significant impact on Patterson and Illig, who strove to incorporate them into their own business philosophy.

Cliff Illig acknowledged that Kauffman's imprint is deeply rooted in *Cerner* culture, and he recalled how quickly Patterson put Kauffman's ideas into practice at the company. "I had an opportunity to spend some quality time with Ewing Kauffman," Illig said, "and I distinctly remember Neal coming back from those meetings just chock-full of some of Mr. K's wisdom. It took just minutes to actually turn some of those thoughts into big actions that have impacted *Cerner* ever since."[14]

One of the principal ways in which Patterson and Illig incorporated Kauffman's first rule, to treat others as you would like to be treated, is through their attitudes toward the people who work for and with the company. Kauffman believed that a strong company does not create a hierarchy of employees who fit into "superior-subordinate relationships."[15] Rather, the company appoints "associates" who work together, with everyone from the manager to the new hire considered equally important to the mission of the company.

"[Kauffman] believed that if associates were treated with dignity and respect that they, too, would treat others, particularly customers and vendors, the same way," Morgan wrote.[16]

Patterson instituted this terminology at *Cerner*. "At *Cerner*, the word 'associate' is used," noted Mike Herman, former president and chief operating officer for the Kauffman Foundation and a member of *Cerner*'s board of directors. *Cerner*'s founders learned how to "treat [their] associates and [their] customers and suppliers with respect, and listen to them and respond to their needs, not [their own] needs."[17]

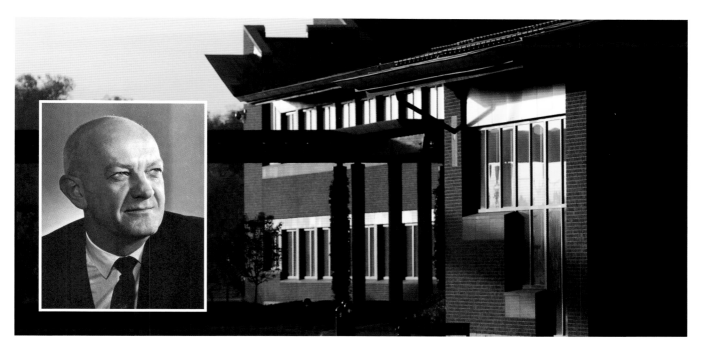

The Ewing Marion Kauffman Foundation, headquartered in Kansas City, serves as a catalyst for entrepreneurial success and innovation in business and education. *(Photography by Dan White. © 2004 Ewing Marion Kauffman Foundation. Used with permission. All rights reserved.)*

Inset: Kauffman, a legendary businessman and philanthropist, established the pharmaceutical giant Marion Laboratories in 1950. *(Photograph courtesy of Ewing Marion Kauffman Foundation. Used with permission. All rights reserved.)*

Another component of the egalitarian culture at *Cerner* is a tradition of Town Hall Meetings, conducted several times a year, in which Patterson joins with all of the associates to discuss the company's activities. Associates in regional offices throughout the country participate in these meetings via satellite broadcast.

Cerner's Town Hall Meetings recall meetings at Marion where associates first gathered around a table after work to share ideas. When the company grew, Kauffman stood on the loading dock to talk with associates about the company highlights and the goals and innovations that would keep Marion on the cutting edge. Eventually these meetings had to take place in an auditorium to accommodate the entire Marion workforce. Part pep rally, part motivational session, these "Marion on the Move" gatherings set the tone for the company and kept the lines of communication open.

"Neal and Cliff understand the importance of keeping in touch with associates," said Carl J. Schramm, Kauffman Foundation president and CEO. "As the company grew, they've used their Town Hall Meetings to take up communication with all the associates to talk about what's going on, and the challenges and opportunities ahead."[18]

Another example of how *Cerner* maintains a non-hierarchical culture is its style of associate badges. Rather than identifying the associate's rank or the department in which the associate works, badges are color-coded to reflect the number of years he or she has been with the company.

This reflects *Cerner*'s knowledge-based community, which values experience over position. Badge colors allow associates to identify others who have the experience to help them solve a problem. The first color code is a red stripe on an ordinary white badge, indicating that an associate has been at the company two years or longer. Next comes a beige badge for those with more than five years at the company.

"New people were always looking for people to act as mentors, someone they could ask a question of," explained Rick Fiske, *Cerner*'s vice president of Classic operations. "So the color-coding was really designed to let people know who had been here a long time." At 10 years, the company added a blue badge, at 15 a green badge, and at 20 a gold badge. "We did things subtly to try to get visual cues for people to recognize knowledge experts and to recognize process experts," Fiske said. "And [we had an] open-door policy. Everyone was [on a] first-name basis."[19]

Cerner incorporated the second tenet of Kauffman's philosophy, sharing the rewards, by carefully developing a program of raises and bonuses. "Mr. Kauffman found out that people want to be treated fairly, not necessarily to be the highest-paid person, and *Cerner* is very diligent, as Marion was, on … giving raises and bonuses based on measurable [performance goals]," Herman explained.[20]

Following Kauffman's third tenet, to give back to the community, *Cerner* has made it a priority to remain actively involved in local civic organizations and schools. The company was an early participant in the North Kansas City School District's School-to-Career Partnership Program, which helps students obtain firsthand awareness of the knowledge, skills, educational requirements, and attitudes necessary for various occupations. The goal of the program is to educate schools about local industries so that the schools could, in turn, provide students with more specialized skills to help them find jobs in those industries.[21]

The company and its associates also established the First Hand Foundation, which provides financially needy children throughout the world with quality medical care. As *Cerner* grew even larger, it continued to reflect the Kauffman philosophy that had formed the company culture from the beginning. Patterson and Illig recognized the value of Kauffman's ideas and the positive effect they had on his own business.

"Mr. K's philosophies and values not only created a positive and productive environment in which to work, but also a profitable company, which created many jobs and great wealth while contributing to the availability of life-saving pharmaceuticals," Morgan wrote.[22]

And *Cerner*, in turn, continued to create jobs not only in Kansas City, but in regional offices throughout the country and the world. And, like Kauffman's company, *Cerner*'s mission was to make a valuable contribution to healthcare.

The Best and the Brightest

In its recruitment materials, *Cerner* points out that a career with the company is more than a job, it's an opportunity to leave a legacy through an organization that is revolutionizing healthcare.

According to one recruiting document, "At the end of the day, *Cerner* associates know that their work makes a difference in the way healthcare is delivered to their families and communities."[23]

Early on, Patterson communicated the message that working at *Cerner* was more of a calling than a way to make a living by identifying the profound role that information technology would take in the medical industry.

"We had found our niche in the world of business, moreover in an industry in which information played not just a big role but *the biggest* role imag-

From left to right: Founders Cliff Illig, Paul Gorup, and Neal Patterson—shown here at a Town Hall Meeting—believe in rewarding associates through performance-based compensation and giving back to the community by remaining actively involved with a variety of organizations.

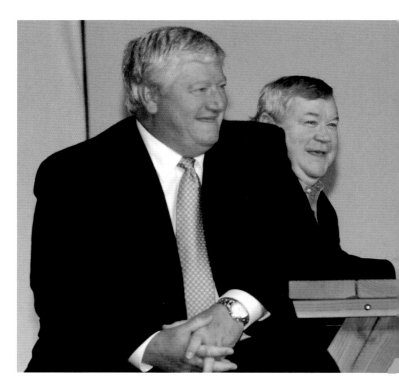

inable in our society—it was a matter of life and death," he said.[24]

This message took hold with recruits such as Liane Lance, the med-tech who began working with Patterson at the MAWD lab in 1979 and advanced to the level of vice president at *Cerner*. "Everything we do is for the betterment of human life," she said in 2004.[25]

The type of associate *Cerner* seeks out is not only attracted to *Cerner*'s mission, but also has the ability to focus intensely on helping push the vision forward. According to Gail Blanchard, who joined *Cerner* in 1987 and became vice president of client organization and leadership, the typical *Cerner* associate is "an overachiever, a self-starter, someone who is self-motivated, someone who is not resistant to handling details and being very focused."[26]

In order to work effectively with associates throughout the company and with the clients they will serve, potential associates also need to be "very personable, able to communicate with people, and be sensitive to a situation," Blanchard added. "Because in a client situation, they're going to have to deal with a whole lot of stuff. You can't let your prejudices or your personality or your style ... get in the way of the message."[27]

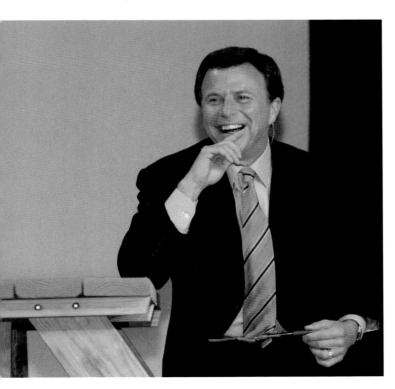

In addition to being a "people person" and possessing outstanding skills, the associate also has to be enthusiastic about learning—constant, in-depth learning. "They need to be aggressive pursuers of knowledge because there's a lot to learn here," Blanchard said.[28]

New associates are also selected for their potential in working with other dedicated and highly motivated people. "There's almost not room for just average people," said Debbie Yantis, vice president of *Cerner* Great Lakes, "because when you're working in big team-based environments and you're working on things collaboratively, if someone doesn't have the work ethic or the commitment ... of others, they just don't feel part of the group. I don't know how to explain it, but that's why I went to work at *Cerner*."[29]

The commitment of *Cerner* associates is rewarded in many ways, including the opportunity to directly contribute to better healthcare for people throughout the world.

"In terms of family and loved ones, there is a personal aspect to enhancing healthcare," said Seth Rupp, one of *Cerner*'s client relationship executives. "The real value proposition is through improving electronic records in relation to efficiencies, reminders, and the consistency of data. There is a significant advantage in that the data from the systems has been up for so long. It has allowed our clients to benefit from the depth and breadth of the applications, as well as from the subsequent data itself."[30]

Mike Neal, vice president of *Cerner* West Services, affirmed the personal rewards of working for the company. "I think the real difference at *Cerner* is what we do with our clients ends up being very personal and passionate. You can't implement solutions within a healthcare environment and not feel very, very connected with the results of what we're trying to achieve. We're not implementing solutions just to help a major Fortune 500 company make more money. We're implementing solutions that really make a difference in our communities, and that touches each of us."[31]

Whether hired at the executive level or advanced during their tenure with the company, *Cerner* executives enjoy a great deal of autonomy. "Neal and Cliff have always hired independent individuals that work well as a team and work well individually," said

Francie McNair-Stoner, vice president of client operations. "They are inspirational in themselves, in that they can get an idea, a big picture across and get a big team motivated to go do beyond what's being asked for today. There's a reporting mechanism to say, here's what we're going to go do, but then you're given the autonomy to go figure out how to best accomplish that."[32]

Cerner's style of executive autonomy has been observed from outside the company as well. "One thing I'm impressed about in *Cerner*'s organization and culture is that employees are given a great deal of latitude and responsibility and accountability and left alone," said Betsy Solberg, executive vice-president of Fleishman-Hillard, Inc., a public relations firm. "I give a lot of talks and I tell young people, 'There are three things you want to do. Find yourself a company that's ethical and that's honest. Find a company that cares about its people and one that is rapidly growing, and that's all you need because if you join a rapidly growing company, that means they have smart people. The company will keep growing and you will be intellectually challenged every day. When you put your feet on the floor in the morning, you can say, "I am going to a great job, a great company that challenges me every morning."' That's what *Cerner* does."[33]

Alan Dietrich, who joined the company in 1990 as director of business planning and development (later called marketing), recalled that his rise through the company was inspired by his mentor, CEO Neal Patterson. "He invested quite a bit in me then in terms of my professional development and my career at *Cerner*. In our annual reviews, the things that he said to me about areas that I needed to work on were surprisingly deep, and I still carry those things with me today. I mean, I can still remember those statements. They weren't said in a disparaging or damaging way; it was [about] 'If you want to be a CEO some day, if you want to head a company some day, you need to work on these three areas,' and great insights, stuff that I hadn't heard from anybody else anywhere, and I respect that a lot."[34]

Vice President and Chief People Officer Julie Wilson was also influenced by this dynamic environment when she began her career with *Cerner* 15 years ago as a contract administrator. After a brief sabbatical to develop a startup organization, Wilson returned to *Cerner*, working in a wide range of positions from managing a small human resources team to overseeing *Cerner*'s extensive properties and facilities.

"I'm going to give credit to Cliff and Neal because they have a very strong interest in ensuring that we have a culture that people want to be a part of, for one thing," said Wilson. "Our culture positions you to have a positive impact on our clients and ... to leave an imprint on society and the way healthcare runs around the world. It's very important; they want this to be a knowledge-driven, high-energy, high-quality, fun, results-oriented kind of environment, and I think that's what it is."[35]

Those who fit well into the *Cerner* culture thrive on this autonomy, as well as on the constant influx of new challenges. "About every year or so, you end up bouncing to something new, and that's the quickest way to grow," said Mike Nill, vice president for technical architecture/operations. "Get thrown into something you're uncomfortable with, and you'll figure out how to be successful."[36]

All of the hiring criteria are geared toward developing and maintaining the unique *Cerner* culture. Patterson always looks for associates who have the capacity for creative thinking and problem solving, and he has learned that it is his job to have faith in associates' abilities and then get out of their way. "It's a matter of trust," he said.[37] Patterson admitted that he had at times been tempted to micromanage, thinking he had a better idea and not delegating a task to an associate. But he learned that this type of management wipes out opportunities for new talent to find a fresh, and possibly better, approach.

"When you start telling someone what to do, you block their new path, the creative innovation that that person can do," he said. The best way to encourage innovation, he said, is to create an environment that brings out the best in people. "You empower from the top. You really trust people, and you just hire bright, energetic people."[38]

Several associates who joined *Cerner* in its early years recalled the passionate commitment to revolutionizing healthcare that the founders expressed in their interviews. Blanchard came to *Cerner* after working for several years at Rubicon, a *Cerner* competitor.

"One of the reasons I left there was that I was not happy with the way they ran the business," she said. "They had a very good product and very good people, but the leadership didn't have a good plan, didn't have good direction, and didn't have vision. They were very shortsighted, and it just didn't seem like a place that was going to be a good place to be for the long run."[39]

When she interviewed at *Cerner* in late 1986, she realized she had found a company that demonstrated the qualities she was looking for. She had been ready to leave the medical IT sector if necessary, but *Cerner* gave her many reasons to stay in the field.

"I just wanted to get to an organization that had the right values, the right ethics, the right direction, and the right culture for me," she said.[40]

Blanchard was impressed by the plans that Patterson, Gorup, Illig, and the other executives described during her visit, goals that reached far beyond the lab setting with which she was very familiar.

"It was striking to me to hear them talk about their vision," she said. "They were a lab company." However, they had well-laid plans for much more, as she learned throughout the interview process. Blanchard recalled:

Cliff and Neal were talking about how the lab is the core of healthcare, and it's going to grow, that what healthcare needs is to expand and have a system that covers the entire patient's medical record.... They had a consistent plan. Everybody that I talked to had the same ... vision in mind.

As I reflected back on my visit, I was very impressed with the people, and I was very impressed with their vision, and I thought, even if they don't hit their vision, it's a great place to be, and they're bound to get closer to that vision than if they didn't have one. It was exciting to be able to stay in the industry and find an organization that you could believe in and feel good about.

After I was [there] for five years, [I remembered that] they had told me about their five-year plan, and we had more than done what was in their five-year plan. Each year, they'd talk about the vision and extending that and [we] would always hit the [mark].[41]

Blanchard, who fit the overachieving, highly motivated profile of a *Cerner* associate, has lived out that enthusiasm and dedication throughout her career. "My life at *Cerner* has been very, very intense," she reflected. "I don't do anything part-

way. If I'm going to do it, we're going to absolutely do it 1,000 percent."[42]

Vice President of Engineering Owen Straub was hired a few months earlier than Blanchard in mid-1986. He had just graduated from Northwest Missouri State University, where he had heard a lot about *Cerner* at recruitment sessions. He hoped to get a job in Kansas City, his hometown, and spoke with Charlie Whitcraft, who was in charge of *Cerner's* engineering team at the time. He was surprised that Whitcraft invited him to come to the office on a Saturday for their initial talk.

Straub had heard that *Cerner* was working on a lab system but had big plans for other clinical systems. He recalled:

The lab was the only solution they had, but they seemed very passionate about it. It's easy for people to talk passionately, but it started becoming pretty visible to me from my first encounter on campus when I came in on a Saturday, and not only was Charlie [there], but there were other people [there]. They seemed very excited. They knew where they wanted it to be, and they were working hard to get there. This was very intriguing to me because I had talked to some other companies, insurance companies and stuff, and they just didn't have the same enthusiasm that I experienced at Cerner.

After I talked to Charlie, I came back in and interviewed with some other people, and at the time, Cerner was still small. So I actually talked to Cliff Illig as one of my interviews for an entry-level position.... I thought, "Wow, this is a growing company. The founders are very interested in the quality of people. That demonstrates that they really want the right people to come in." I just wasn't experiencing that same kind of feeling at other places I was interviewing, and that really intrigued me.[43]

Cerner's passion for its vision did not wane during the next decade. Dick Flanigan, who joined the company as a sales manager in 1994, was attracted by the same visionary enthusiasm and attitude that had been expressed to recruits in the early 1980s.

He had been working for a major *Cerner* competitor, IBM, as manager of its Healthcare Business Unit, when a former IBM executive, Trace Devanny, asked him to take a look at *Cerner*. Devanny had left IBM to become *Cerner's* regional vice president for the Mid-Atlantic region in the spring of 1994, and he was anxious to introduce Flanigan to the company. Flanigan wasn't looking for a move, however.

"Frankly, if I was going to leave IBM, I wasn't going to go be a sales manager for somebody else," he said. "That wasn't a career move I wanted. So moving to Kansas City was not really a thought, but Trace invited me to come out, and I was more than intrigued on my visit. I thought, 'This place is actually pretty cool.'" Flanigan continued:

I would say the first thing [that impressed me] was that I really perceived they were clinically focused as a company.... It was very impressive to me that Cerner had a core understanding of what it took to deliver patient care, and I was impressed that the people that I met were consistently talking about the vision and talking about healthcare at a healthcare level, not at a technology level. So it was very intriguing from that perspective, that it was a healthcare company that sold software....

Secondly, IBM has really good people. IBM has been hiring from the top 1 percent of the gene pool for 70 years. So I had this view that if I went to this small company, there's no way I'm going to be working with good people. I mean, I know Trace. He's a good guy, but I really thought there was going to be this big step down in the quality of the people when I got there. I was blown away [to find that] these are actually some really good people.[44]

One of those "really good people" was Doug Krebs, a former director at IBM who became president of *Cerner* Global.

"Doug is a few years older than I am," Flanigan said, "but he moved up through the corporation pretty quickly, and I kept thinking, 'Why would Doug Krebs leave IBM? He was going places.' That really intrigued me."[45]

Finally, Flanigan was inspired by the infectious enthusiasm and clear direction at *Cerner*. "I thought this was a more entrepreneurial, just a much more exciting, make-your-way kind of company," he said.[46]

Work Hard/Play Hard

"In the early days, we always worked Saturday," said Kim Stevens, who joined *Cerner* as Neal Patterson's administrative assistant in 1986. "If you

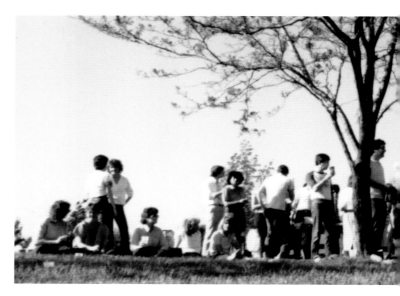

were not there, you were truly missed, and everyone wondered what you were up to."[47]

Long hours in the office and long weeks on the road were common for most associates, but camaraderie was strong, and they enjoyed spending a few off hours together, as well. A tradition of "Beer Fridays" began the year Stevens began her 12-year career at *Cerner*.

"On May 1, 1986, we decided to have a May Day party. It was a Friday.... The whole company played baseball together in the afternoon. That Saturday, Cliff said, 'That was a lot of fun. We should do it every Friday.'"[48] After that, associates began rolling out a keg of beer from the copy room every Friday afternoon at 4 P.M. sharp.

"Every three weeks we'd go through a keg," Stevens said. "As we grew, it became every two. People would stay until about six o'clock. We also always had soft drinks. At the gathering place around the keg, you'd hear about everyone's travels for the week, the projects they were working on."[49]

That May Day baseball game was also the start of a sports tradition at the company. Associates enjoyed each other's company and, in many cases, considered their co-workers extended family. "We were very much into sports—basketball, baseball, volleyball," Stevens said. "Even after we had kids, we continued to do things together. We held company picnics on a regular basis. It was fun to interact with each other's families."[50]

In 1989, *Cerner* associates took their hard-playing attitude to a new level by participating for the first

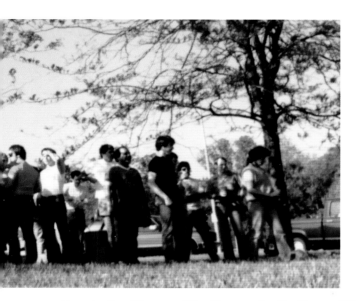
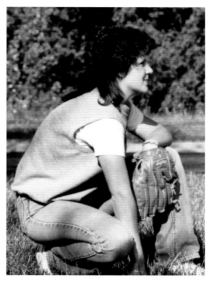
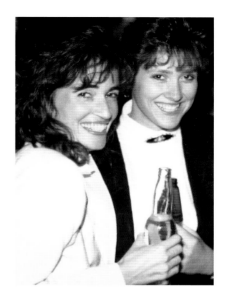

time in the Kansas City Corporate Challenge (KCCC), a highly competitive sports event held every May and June. Launched in 1980 as the first competition of its kind in the nation, the KCCC is designed as an Olympic-styled event that aims to promote fitness and recreation within the city's business community.

The event has grown exponentially every year to become one of the biggest corporate sporting events in the nation. In 2003, 20,000 individuals from 164 companies participated in competitions that included track events, swimming, tennis, racquetball, basketball, billiards, soccer, golf, and biking. Each year, money from corporate entry fees is donated to a charity in the community.

Cerner hit the KCCC running its first year, missing first place by just 0.2 points. For the next 10 years, from 1990 to 1999, *Cerner* took first place at the games. Due to an increase in the number of associates, the company then moved up to the A Division and even more intense competition. It fell short of a win in 2000 and 2001, but made a comeback in 2002. Mark Brewer, a software architect at *Cerner* since 1993, has participated in most of the games during his career with the company. He now wears a *Cerner* logo tattoo on his ankle, a product of a KCCC incentive for team members to do their best. Brewer explained:

> *After the 1999 Challenge, like Michael Jordan and a plethora of other athletes better than myself, I retired, then came back from retirement to coordinate* Cerner's *efforts in the KCCC in*

Above left: The first May Day baseball game led to competitions in other sports, including basketball, volleyball, and eventually the Kansas City Corporate Challenge.

Above center: The *Cerner* traditions of sports competitions and Beer Fridays began on May 1, 1986, when associates gathered outside for a May Day party.

Above right: Beer Fridays are a longstanding tradition at *Cerner*. The late afternoon get-togethers allow associates to recharge after a week of long hours at the office and many miles on the road.

Below: From left to right, current Chief of Staff Jeff Townsend and former associates Paul Evans and Paul Pearce socialize at a company picnic in 1986. The company's work hard/play hard philosophy manifests itself with regular picnics, where associates enjoy interacting with each other's families.

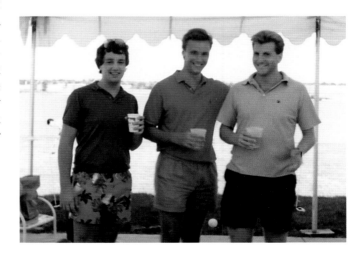

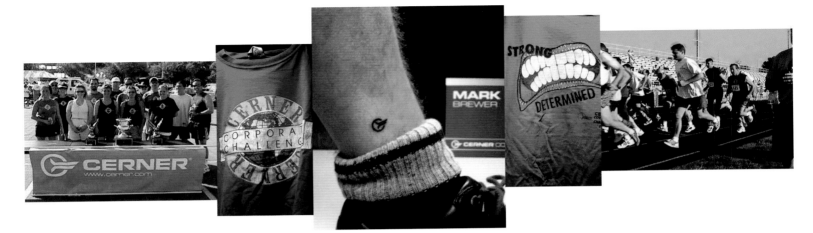

2002. [Senior Project Leader] Jennifer Kultala-Smith and I were approached—begged—to come out of retirement and coordinate in 2002. With a host of other incentives for participation, we came up with the incentive to "Tattoo Brew" with the Cerner logo if we won in Division A. We won by three points [and I] fulfill[ed] my promise to my fellow associates.[51]

In 2003, *Cerner* came in third place in Division A, with 80 associates competing against employees from 15 Kansas City companies who participated in that division. Division A stand-outs included much larger companies Hallmark and Sprint, which took first and second place, respectively. Many *Cerner* associates continued to train year-round in preparation for upcoming games, as well as to enjoy the health benefits of exercise.

Learning Curve

In an industry as complex as medical IT, associate and client training is as crucial to success as the quality of the solution itself. *Cerner*'s associate training program evolved into a standardized, comprehensive strategy in the late 1990s, but prior to that, most programs fell short of what associates required.

The company committed itself to a strong associate training program in 1996 with the hiring of Robert Campbell, a learning and development professional who had worked for Arthur Andersen for a number of years before moving on

Above, from left to right: A winning *Cerner* team after the 2002 Kansas City Corporate Challenge; a T-shirt from the 1994 KCCC; Associate Mark Brewer's *Cerner* tattoo, celebrating the company's Division A win in 2002; the back of the 1994 T-shirt, which reads, "strong, determined, fast;" and *Cerner* team members (in white T-shirts) competing in a 2004 track event.

Below: A case in the entryway of the Associate Center displays trophies won by *Cerner* teams in the Kansas City Corporate Challenge. *(Photo by Antonia Felix.)*

to AT&T. In his first talks with *Cerner* executives, Campbell got a clear picture of the company's needs.

Campbell learned that training was inconsistent because each team had its own approach. In many cases, associates only received a brief introduction to solutions that did not prepare them adequately for presenting these complex systems to clients. The process was more like a harrowing sink-or-swim experience that did not serve anyone well.

"There were cases," Campbell said, "where we would literally hire someone on a Monday [and] have them go through the paperwork. On ... Wednesday, we'd introduce them to an application.... They'd kind of run through it. In some cases, they'd be out in front of a client ... presenting or discussing that application on ... Friday of that same week. Honest to goodness, in some cases, actually doing that solo, on their own. That just wasn't good for the associate or the client."[52]

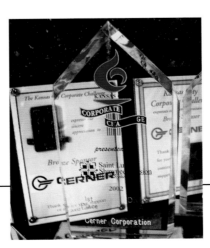

In 1995, one year before Campbell's arrival, leaders of various departments had responded to the need for a more standardized approach to training with a company-wide program called Traditions. This module gave new associates a big-picture view of the company with sessions on *Cerner's* history, culture, vision, and organizational structure. From its overview of company history to "how-to" sessions about software development, marketing, and other aspects of the business, Traditions played an integral part in creating *Cerner's* culture.

Illig talked to associates about company philosophy in a session called "The *Cerner* Approach," offering an overview of the company's core values. He told associates that the company could envision, create, design, and build the most functional, sophisticated IT system in the world, but that it takes people—extraordinary associates—to make it work. The company's goal to "exceed client expectations" would be fulfilled by a strategy of working through "courteous aggressive action." The effects of this philosophy, according to Illig's presentation, are defined by *Cerner's* concept of the "magic moment"—"a split second in time when you have amazed, delighted, surprised, and exceeded all expectations with an act or gesture."[53]

Illig also drew upon Walt Disney Company CEO Michael Eisner's statement that, "Our front line equals our bottom line" to explain that at *Cerner*, the bottom line consists of two factors: the front line and the client relationship. In this scenario, *Cerner* executives work for the front line. Illig added that associates should continually keep this philosophy in mind by reminding themselves, "If I'm not doing things to further [the company], I should not be working here."[54]

This standardized approach had been lacking in the training that each team had developed on its own. Although there were some teams that did fairly well, the training was not consistent, and Traditions was the first answer to that challenge. *Cerner* had also held one Associate Conference, in which the company essentially shut down for one week with all associates gathering for a centralized training conference.

The company's executives knew that more was needed, however, and during Campbell's final interview for the job, he and Patterson had an intense debate at the CEO's home on how best to improve associate education. A glimpse at their discussion gives insight into Patterson's style and approach not only to hiring, but to problem-solving.

Campbell was actually very happy with his current position at AT&T, which gave him an open, nothing-to-lose attitude going into the *Cerner* interview process, and after his first round of interviews he had been told he had the job. Then, a week later, he got a call informing him that Patterson wanted to talk to him first.

Campbell chalked the confusion up to the dynamic of the company. "I think that's kind of indicative of the kind of company *Cerner* is, right? It was young, fast-growing, entrepreneurial. Kind of, every day is a new day." Campbell described his interview with Patterson:

> I met with Neal, and we spent a good two or three hours just talking about learning and development, the role it plays in an organization, what we needed to accomplish broadly at Cerner.... It was a pretty vigorous debate at some points in that dialogue. We disagreed on some points, but came to agreement on most points. But there was absolutely no intimidation or reluctance to speak my mind because, again, I was very secure in what I was doing. I wasn't necessarily looking for a new job opportunity.
>
> He responded really well to that, and it was probably one of the most challenging and engaging discussions I've had on the topic of learning and development. I found Neal to be well-versed and well-read. He understood the field well. So after about two hours of this, he pulled out a blank sheet of paper and set it on the table. He said, "OK, Rob, I think we're on the same page in terms of our view of what needs to happen here. Let's design it. What should it look like? What should our learning and development function at Cerner look like? You're the guy to lead it. Let's do it."
>
> It's just really invigorating to be sitting down with the CEO of the company and have that kind of an experience before you come in the door.[55]

The ideas on the page that Patterson and Campbell drew up during their first meeting involved developing programs around clients, associates, and business partners and "making sure that we understood that each of those audiences was unique and important," Campbell said.[56]

The second major component of the design was to incorporate a system of knowledge flow throughout the organization. They realized that they needed to create a way to capture knowledge and codify it in a way that would make it available to those who needed it. This was a challenge for *Cerner*.

"In a young, entrepreneurial company, you've got a bunch of cowboys," Campbell said. "Everyone is doing things their own way. There's a lot of prestige to being the expert, right?"[57]

Cerner went on to develop a comprehensive training process known as Compass. All associates began their *Cerner* careers with the one-week Compass: Destination Transformation orientation program at company headquarters in North Kansas City. The first part of the orientation was a broader version of the Traditions program that introduced associates to the overall culture and structure of the company.

The second segment, Getting Started, helped associates become familiar with *Cerner*'s associate desktop system. Sessions included hands-on tutorials on laptop computers that each associate used. Associates also took classes that discussed *Cerner*'s philosophies (work hard/play hard), code of conduct (security and confidentiality), dress code (no denim), and other practical concerns.

After the orientation, associates began a training program that was tailored to their specific job.

In addition to job-specific training, associates began working with their managers on an in-depth career development plan. Ongoing development and advancement is a priority, and *Cerner* promotes continuing education through tuition reimbursement, professional certification reimbursement, professional affiliation sponsorships, scholarships, and a job-posting service called the Career Navigation Center.

Cerner's high standards for new associates are part of the leadership philosophy that have brought the company to the pinnacle of the medical IT industry.

As articulated in *Cerner*'s 1996 annual report, published when the company had launched its new commitment to associate training, the driving force of good leadership is a combination of people and vision. "The power of an organization," the report stated, "lies in its ability to combine the talents and dreams of many individuals, all contributing to a common vision and strategy, with a goal of providing outstanding benefits for the clients it serves."[58]

Expanding on this idea, the report continued:

> *Cerner's leadership combines the strength of dedicated, long-tenured executives who shaped the corporation, with the fresh insights of less-tenured but talented individuals who offer their industry and technology expertise. Together, they lead the organization with a combination of vision, experience, perseverance, flexibility, commitment, and dependability, a combination that allows us to meet the dynamic needs of the health industry.*[59]

The following year, the company acknowledged the challenges of attracting the top-level talent it

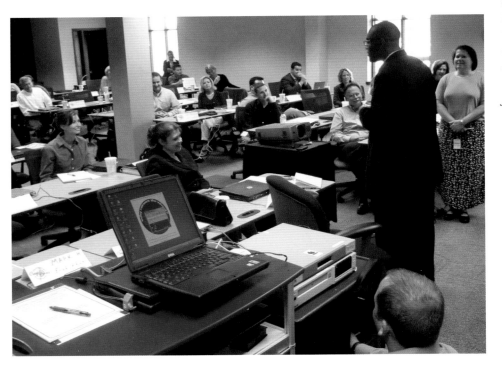

Associates participate in the company's one-week Compass training program, which includes an orientation session, a Traditions segment on *Cerner* culture and structure, as well as classes tailored to specific roles.

needed to succeed in the software industry. "There is a major shortage of software engineers in this country," the 1997 annual report stated. "As it is for most information technology companies, this shortage is a major threat to *Cerner*'s long-term success. A significant indicator of our future competitiveness is our success in attracting top talent from college campuses."[60]

The company was pleased with its recruitment rate and reported that it succeeded in hiring 65 percent of engineers who were offered positions. The company regularly recruited on about 60 campuses throughout the country, making offers to the top students in each class. During the industry boom during that time, those students typically had offers from at least 10 other companies.

As future national awards would reveal, *Cerner*'s success in acquiring top talent was largely due to the progressive culture it so carefully developed.

In addition to software designers and other technical specialists, *Cerner* has hired large numbers of healthcare clinicians throughout its history. These professionals play vital roles in the development of *Cerner* solutions, as well as in other facets of the company. As of March 2005, the company employed nearly 1,000 clinicians from several facets of medicine including M.D.s, R.N.s, clinical Ph.D.s, lab technicians, radiation technicians, pharmacists, health managers and administrators, and medical technicians.

These professionals "have decided now to take part of their career into bringing technology and solutions to help change workflow and process to improve patient safety, reduce expense, and get waste out of the system," said Paul Sinclair, senior vice president of *Cerner* Great Lakes Services.[61]

The "Hotline" and Other Commitments to Service

Cerner recognized early that client support and training had been neglected in the medical IT industry and vowed to change that. In 1985, the company established a 24-hour-a-day/7-day-a-week Immediate Response service that, at the time, was a revolutionary concept.

According to Rick Fiske:

At that time in the industry, if you called for a service point in the middle of the night, you

THE D³ BLOOPER

WHEN *CERNER* SOFTWARE ENGIneers began to work on a new base architecture for *Cerner* solutions, they used several different terms for it, including Tablerock, V or Version 500, and *Cerner* Millennium.

One working title that stuck, at least for a little while, was D³, a term that reflected the directory layouts they were working with.

After using the name for about three weeks, some of the clinical personnel associated with the project heard about it and informed *Cerner* engineers and marketing staff that D³ was shorthand for the medical term *decubitus*, or bedsores.

"The nurses were going, 'D³—bedsores— we can't do that!'" recalled engineer Owen Straub. "We realized that we probably needed to expand our audience in naming. If we left it up to engineering to name it, we probably would have called it something really weird."[1]

got an answering service. Traditionally, [the service] called somebody at their home, woke them up, and tried to figure out how to support the client. Remember, you're talking pre-Internet, high-volume, pre-cable TV, DSL lines—dial-up modems at best. That whole service side didn't work.

We started our Immediate Response in 1985. We actually called it "the hotline" at that time. It was seven days a week, 24 hours a day, never shut down. ... It was totally new. Suddenly when the phone answered, it was a real person whose only job was to fix the client's problem.[62]

The new hotline, a telephone ER for client emergencies, was part of *Cerner*'s goal to consistently exceed clients' expectations. Another was its team approach to client service, a strategy the com-

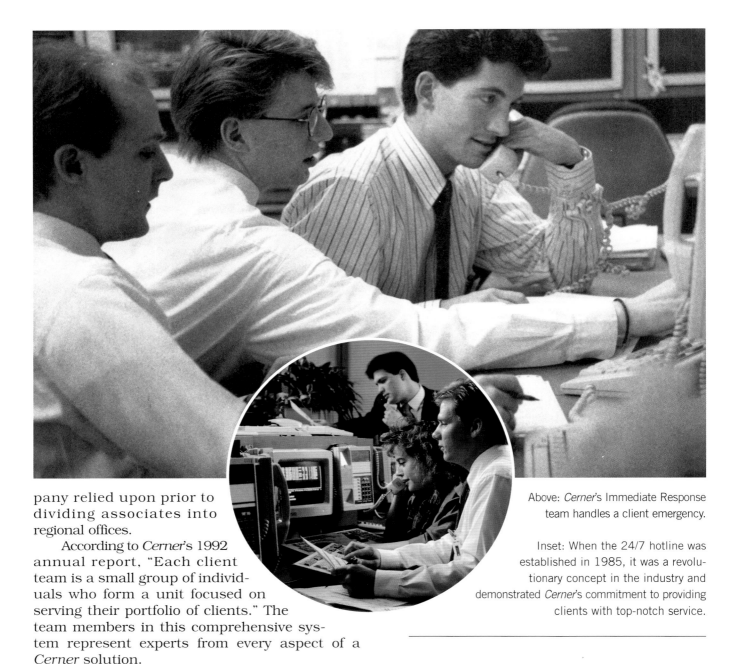

Above: *Cerner*'s Immediate Response team handles a client emergency.

Inset: When the 24/7 hotline was established in 1985, it was a revolutionary concept in the industry and demonstrated *Cerner*'s commitment to providing clients with top-notch service.

pany relied upon prior to dividing associates into regional offices.

According to *Cerner*'s 1992 annual report, "Each client team is a small group of individuals who form a unit focused on serving their portfolio of clients." The team members in this comprehensive system represent experts from every aspect of a *Cerner* solution.

"Each team has a project manager to provide leadership and guidance, application analysts to handle the clinical aspects of technical issues, software analysts to troubleshoot technical software concerns, and system analysts to manage our clients' technology issues," the report stated.[63] It explained that even in this "Age of Service," the concept of strategic partnership with clients, such as *Cerner*'s client-team approach, was "foreign to many business enterprises."

Another groundbreaking development in client service occurred in 1986 with the launch of the annual *Cerner* Health Conference (CHC). This symposium, attended by 35 clients, featured detailed introductions to *Cerner* solutions and was created to give clients the benefit of talking to solution experts in order to achieve one critical goal: the delivery of better patient care.

In its first years, the CHC quickly expanded into a conference that provides educational sessions, interactive exhibits featuring *Cerner* solutions, and nationally known speakers. Participants also gain new insight into the medical IT field through forums, workshops, and discussions with industry experts, technicians, and healthcare executives.

Cerner had decided early on that client service would be one of the primary cornerstones of its overall vision.

According to the company's 1992 annual report, "Just as *Cerner*'s HNA applications weave together the many threads of clinical information, so are client services and associate enrichment woven into the fabric of the company's overall vision and business plan."[64]

The 2004 CHC, held at the Gaylord Palms Resort & Convention Center in Orlando, Florida, was attended by more than 1,900 *Cerner* clients and individual participants. This conference gave partic-

ipants the opportunity to explore the cutting-edge advancements in the industry with *Cerner* exhibits, as well as displays by hundreds of Solutions Gallery exhibitors such as IBM, 3M Healthcare, General Data, and Oracle. The three keynote speakers were Richard Granger, Director-General for the United Kingdom's National Programme for IT; Mark McClellan, M.D., Ph.D., Administrator, Centers for Medicare and Medicaid Services; and *Cerner* CEO Neal Patterson.

CEO Neal Patterson takes the stage during a general session of the 2004 *Cerner* Health Conference in Orlando, Florida. More than 1,900 clients attended the event, which also featured exhibits on advancements in the industry and displays of healthcare IT solutions.

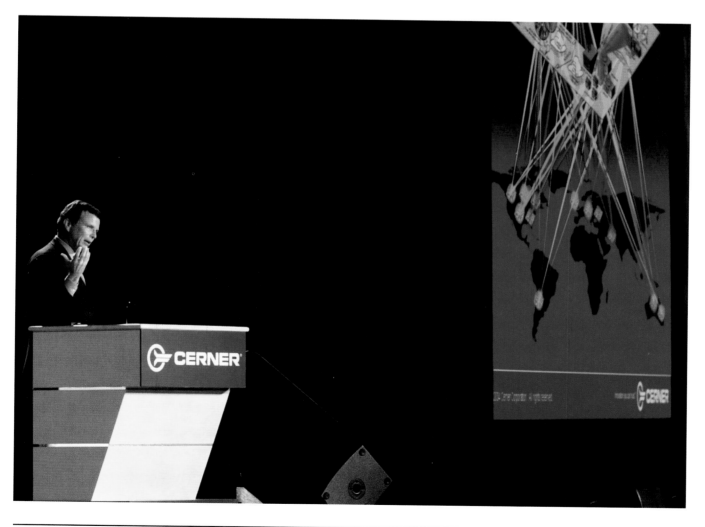

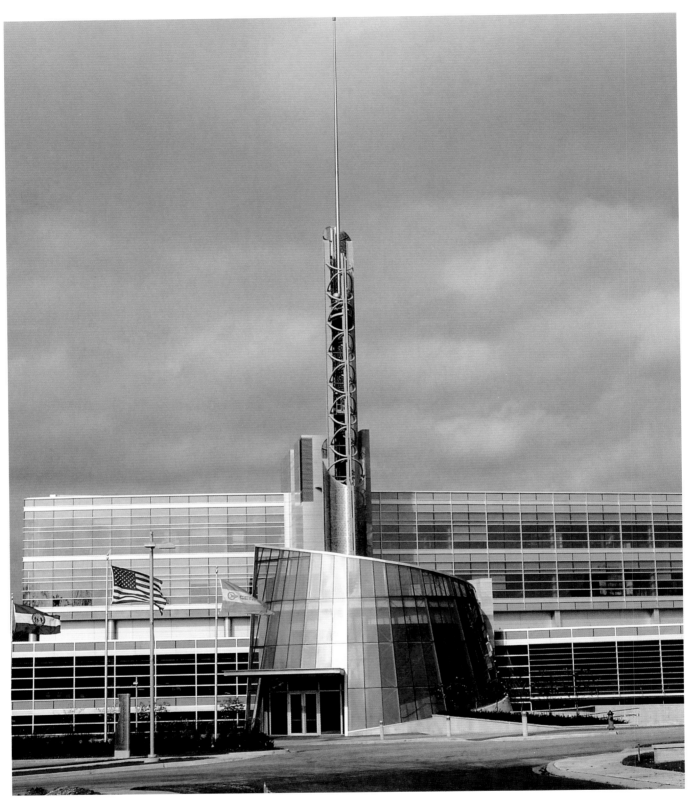

After considering other locations, *Cerner* bought the entire Rockcreek Office Park in 1994, primarily because the property offered plenty of room for expansion. In 2000, the company began a 10-year, $191 million expansion of its World Headquarters, and in the fall of 2003, this ultramodern building connecting 2800 and 2900 Rockcreek Parkway opened. *(Photo by Antonia Felix.)*

CHAPTER FOUR

DESIGNED FOR GROWTH

Our assets are not in [facilities], they're in people's heads.

—Cliff Illig, *Cerner* co-founder[1]

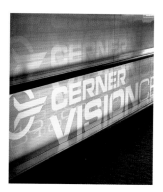

W HEN PGI & ASSOCIATES went into business in 1980, the company leased an office in a small building near the Country Club Plaza just south of downtown Kansas City. With its move to an office park in North Kansas City in 1981, the company embarked on a course of continuous growth that was reflected by a series of expansions at its home base.

Over the years, *Cerner*'s executives took great pride in the transformation of corporate headquarters into a stunning, ultramodern campus. In 2000, *Cerner* launched a 10-year, $191 million expansion of its World Headquarters, the highlight of which was the grand opening in the fall of 2003 of a striking new building designed to visually manifest the company's mission and leadership in medical information technology.

These expansive facilities represent more than just physical assets. They are symbolic of the enduring vision of the company, which continues to grow through regional offices across the globe and has assumed a leading role in the healthcare IT industry.

Breaking New Ground—1981 to 2003

When PGI moved from downtown to North Kansas City in 1981, just across the road from North Kansas City Hospital, the company made a secret statement with its new main phone number.

Hidden in this number, 816-221-1024, was a clue to the company's identity as a technology-based business: there are 1,024 bytes in 1K of file data.[2]

PGI's 25 associates set up shop in 5,000 square feet of office space on the sixth floor of the building at 2800 Rockcreek Parkway, one of six buildings in the office park.[3] Patterson took the southwest corner office—which he still occupies—and Illig and Gorup took the adjoining two window offices on the west side. All of the company's associates worked in cubicles just outside those three offices, which kept the founders in close proximity to their team at all times.

"We worked very, very closely with them," recalled Gay Johannes, who was hired as a programmer in June 1983. "Neal was always looking over our shoulders and saying, 'What are you working on? Where are we at? How are things going?' They were very involved and worked very closely with us on a daily basis. With 20 to 25 people, we were very interactive and worked closely together."[4]

Doctors, dentists, and other businesses such as Union Pacific and CitiCorp also leased space at

The Vision Center, which opened in 1992, allows potential clients to see demonstrations of live code as it would operate in doctors' offices, labs, and nurses' stations. *(Photo by Antonia Felix.)*

the Rockcreek Office Park, but as PGI grew into *Cerner* Corporation, it took over additional space on the sixth floor. Vice President of Engineering Steve Oden, who joined the company in 1985 (as associate No. 81), recalled associates' excitement during those first expansions.

"The big thing is, when we displaced some dentist or physician ... on the far end of this floor and built our training center, we were training [Philadelphia's] Albert Einstein Medical Center and some other clients on [*PathNet®* solution] Anatomic Pathology," he said. "It was a big, big deal when this probably 30-seat classroom opened, and we had a stage and tables."[5]

In this expanded section of the sixth floor, clients were invited to view demonstrations and to partake in training sessions on building the database for their facility's solutions. As the lead engineer, Oden directed that initial training.

Todd Downey, who joined the company as a staff accountant in 1986, was invigorated by the teamwork approach on the sixth floor and impressed by the founders' close interaction with their teams.

"I remember that the first week I was here, I probably worked 65 hours," Downey said. "My roommate at the time—we had both just left Investicore as stockbrokers—wondered what kind of place I had found here. [He wondered], 'What can be so exciting about a place when you're 22 years old that you're going to work 65 hours a week at it?' "[6]

Downey also described the unique working environment in which Cliff Illig—the company's executive vice president, secretary, treasurer, and

---

CERNER DOCTRINE

VISION CENTER

ORIGINALLY OPENED IN 1992, THE Vision Center was expanded in 1995 to include seven presentation rooms and enhanced technology in the central control room, allowing associates to create custom presentations for each client that focus specifically on the solutions they require. The theater and meeting rooms provide high-tech spaces for holding conversations with executives, clinicians, and other professionals involved in putting *Cerner*'s solutions to work at healthcare facilities.

"The Vision Center is, at its essence, about relationship-based selling," explained Chief Marketing Officer Donald Trigg. "That's a way the company has historically brought existing and prospective clients to Kansas City and allowed them to see something, which is very intangible in software, in a much more tangible way."[1]

Cerner's approach to the Vision Center is crucial to *Cerner*'s ability to transform healthcare around the world. The Vision Center experience inspires collaboration, focus, and long-term relationships.

"The Vision Center is the place where we tackle the tough issues facing our industry and work together, with our clients, to solve them," said Andy Heeren, *Cerner* Vision Center program manager.[2]

The foundation that is built in the Vision Center is the first step toward a strategy to impact care within organizations and communities. For the past 25 years, *Cerner* has focused on providing health professionals with the right information at the right time to achieve optional health outcomes. The Vision Center allows that goal to be a reality as it is the place that forms the cornerstone of all *Cerner*'s current and future development.

"We are passionate about creating an experience for our clients and in order to execute consistently and with superior quality, we have extensive standard operating procedures, processes, methodologies, communication standards, etc. that come together to create the seamless experience we craft for all Vision Center guests," summarized Heeren.[3]

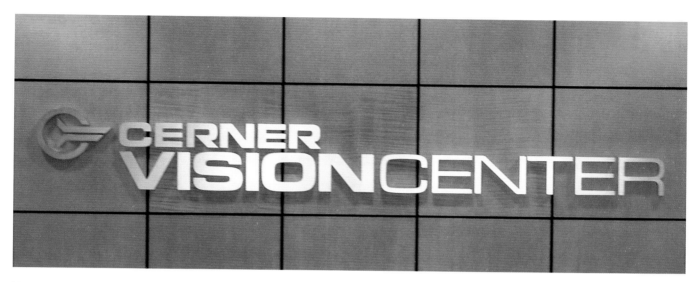

The Vision Center was expanded in 1995 to include seven presentation rooms and enhanced technology that allows associates to create custom demonstrations for each client. (Photo by Antonia Felix.)

director at the time—rolled up his sleeves to work with an entry-level accountant.

"Cliff Illig worked right along next to me at a table for the whole first week," he said. "I thought that was pretty neat, being 22 years old and having the vice president of the company working in the project room with me, digging through binders and contracts."[7]

By 1986, *Cerner* had grown to 149 associates and, with continued growth on the horizon, needed to expand into a bigger space. In October of that year, *Cerner* reported, "The company believes that within the next 18 months it will be required to either lease additional space or acquire or lease a building for its own use."[8]

The company decided to lease more space at Rockcreek, as the location was very well suited for *Cerner* associates and clients. Set on 98 acres of rocky, wooded terrain, less than half of which was developed, the site was a peaceful alternative to downtown and offered easy access to Kansas City International Airport. Another consideration was the fact that approximately 60 percent of *Cerner* associates lived in the Northland, the northern suburbs of Kansas City, which made Rockcreek more convenient. In addition, clients could easily view *PathNet*® solutions at North Kansas City Hospital.

CERNER DOCTRINE
ARCHITECTURE

"**O**NE PATIENT, ONE ARCHITEC-ture," the idea that the patient is at the heart of the healthcare process, is the premise on which *Cerner*'s Healthcare Network Architecture (HNA) was designed.[1] Even a patient with multiple conditions must be related to as a person as a whole, and the care of such a patient is best managed by information technology with a single application architecture.

Like an automobile, a complete clinical information system has many parts: application software, CPUs, memory systems, operating software, a number of layered software products, and networks. Just as most people buy a whole car instead of purchasing various parts from several manufacturers and assembling them haphazardly, it is more practical to implement a single clinical information system founded on a single architecture.

This complete package approach provides a unified design, function, and service for higher quality healthcare.

By the spring of 1990, *Cerner* had grown to 380 associates, and in May the company expanded its office space with a new lease with Leo Eisenberg Company, the firm that managed Rockcreek Office Park. *Cerner* then took up three full floors in the four-story Rockcreek III office building, and the 107,269-square-foot space became the largest business lease to be signed in the Kansas City area that year. The company had been courted by other developers to move into facilities such as Executive Hills North and the University of Missouri-Kansas City's research park, but the many positives of the Rockcreek location persuaded *Cerner* to stay.

By 1993, *Cerner* had more than doubled in size once again. The next year, the company was forced to find accommodations for the more than 600 associates, of more than 1,000 total, dispersed through three office buildings at Rockcreek.

One of the most innovative new additions to the facility during that time was the Vision Center, which opened in 1992 on the second floor of the 2800 building. Designed like a theater, with sets that portray doctors' offices, labs, nurses' stations, and other environments, the center gives new and potential clients an opportunity to view exactly how the solutions would work at their own facilities.

Cerner's expanding office space in the early 1990s coincided with the company's financial growth to $101 million in revenues in 1992, and in January 1994, *Cerner* announced that it would purchase the entire Rockcreek Office Park. The abundance of undeveloped land at the site made it the perfect location for *Cerner*'s ambitious expansion plans. The property featured 409,000 total square feet of office space, with an additional 35 acres available for future building projects.

"We couldn't be constrained any longer," Illig told the *Kansas City Star* in January 1994. "The ability to be able to expand is important to us."[9] According to Patterson, "When we looked at locations, the ability to expand to at least 1 million square feet was an absolute requirement."[10]

Cerner executives had considered other locations, including the downtown Crown Center area, the Briarcliff West development in the Northland, and out-of-state properties in Kansas and other Southern states. Relocating to either coast was never an option, however. By that time, *Cerner* had opened regional offices all over the United States, as well as in Australia, Europe, and other foreign countries, and Kansas City was central to it all.

"We work all over the world and all over this country," Patterson said. "You might as well wake up in the middle of it when you don't know which direction you're going to be going the next day."[11]

Cerner bought the Rockcreek property for approximately $20 million from a group of investors called Northtown Devco. The timing was great for Devco, since one of its major tenants, CitiCorp, was planning to vacate its 60,000 square feet of space at Rockcreek to move into new offices near the airport.

Even though *Cerner* executives had never before considered investing in real estate, buying Rockcreek was much more cost-effective than constructing new headquarters. The deal cost about $49 a square foot, whereas new construction would have cost approximately $100 a square foot.

"It's a good deal for the shareholders," Illig said.[12] Although the company inherited several tenants who would provide rental income, *Cerner*'s priority in buying the property was to build headquarters that could continue to expand with the company. "Our assets are not in [facilities], they're in people's heads," Illig said.

Five years after buying Rockcreek, *Cerner* announced a grand expansion plan that had to be submitted to the North Kansas City Council for a public hearing and approval. The plan called for building nine new buildings on the site over a period of 15 years, which would bring the available office space to Patterson's goal of 1 million square feet.

The expansion would generate $27.3 million in real estate taxes for the city over 25 years, a large increase over the $15.5 million that the existing property would bring in.[13] Part of the agreement with the City Council called for *Cerner* to keep its headquarters in Kansas City, and the council approved *Cerner*'s plans in February 2000.

In addition to approving the $191 million expansion, the city granted *Cerner* $38.8 million in property tax relief under Missouri's Chapter 353 redevelopment law. This tax plan, which applied to the new buildings the company was planning, would allow *Cerner* to forgo paying real estate taxes on the buildings for 10 years, then pay 50 percent of the taxes for 15 years.

The expansion plan called for nine new buildings, each from one to four stories in height, for *Cerner*'s exclusive use, which would increase total office space to 1 million square feet. The plan also called for more than 4,500 spaces in new parking garages and lots. The expansion, to be orchestrated by Kansas City-based architectural firm Gould Evans Goodman Associates, called for five phases of construction to be completed by 2010.

Groundbreaking for the first new building began in July 2001. Situated between two existing buildings, the four-story structure would serve as a welcome center and reflect a new ultramodern, high-tech design for the entire complex. At the time of the groundbreaking ceremony, *Cerner* had grown to 3,400 associates, and executives were confident the company would continue to expand.

"Our confidence in how much we're going to grow over the next 10 years is very, very large," Patterson said at the groundbreaking. "I do believe that this will be a multibillion-dollar company, and I do believe that the number of *Cerner* associates, certainly around the world, will probably hit 10,000."[14]

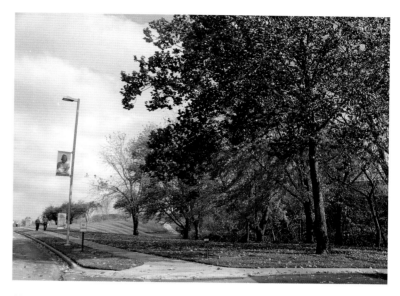

Above: The Rockcreek Office Park, which became *Cerner*'s World Headquarters, is situated on a leafy 98 acres.

Below: The company's Riverport Learning Center, a complex of buildings approximately two miles east of *Cerner* headquarters, opened in April 2002. *(Photos by Antonia Felix.)*

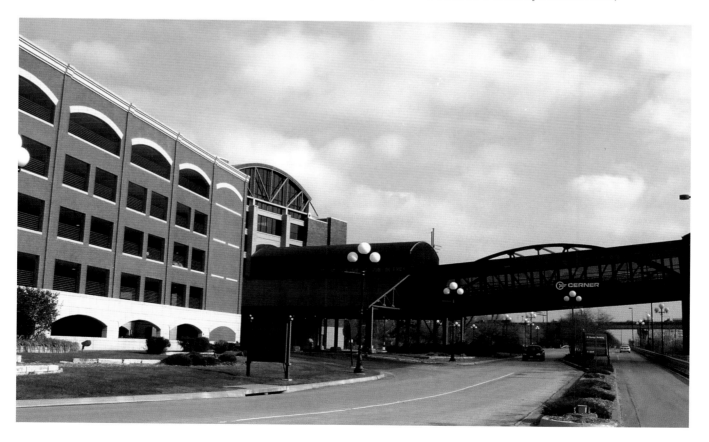

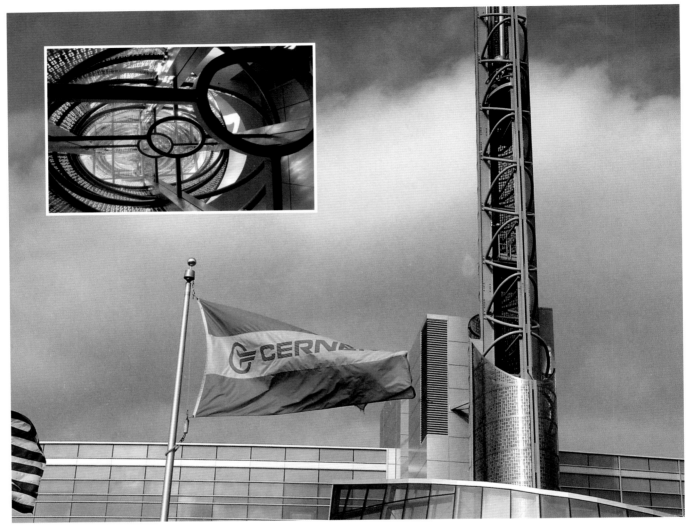

Above: A tower capping the building that connects the 2800 and 2900 Rockcreek Parkway offices was designed to represent strands of human DNA and the zeroes and ones that make up binary computer code. *(Photo by Antonia Felix.)*

Inset: A view from inside the tower.

In addition to the expansion plans at Rockcreek, *Cerner* branched out by leasing 16,000 square feet of office space for a data center at the Summit Technology Campus in Lee's Summit, Missouri, about 24 miles south of North Kansas City. The company took over the high-tech space that had formerly been home to AT&T's microelectronics plant.[15]

The ever-expanding associate training program also needed a new home, and *Cerner* bought a complex of buildings that had formerly been Sam's Town casino, about two miles east of its headquarters on the bank of the Missouri River. *Cerner* paid $4 million for the site and spent another $2 million on renovations, and the new Riverport Learning Center opened in April 2002.[16]

On October 7, 2003, the company celebrated the completion of phase one of the expansion with a dedication ceremony at headquarters. Guest speakers included Missouri Governor Bob Holden and Kansas City Mayor Kay Barnes.

The showpiece of the first phase was a new building that connected the 2800 and 2900 Rockcreek Parkway offices. The 123,500-square-foot building was capped by a 188-foot, stainless-steel tower designed to represent the double helix of human

DNA and the zeroes and ones that make up binary computer code.

"It's the combination of those two that represent the future of healthcare and of medicine," Patterson said at the ceremony.[17]

Inside, the new building featured an auditorium that seats 160 to 165; an expanded Vision Center, where *Cerner* demonstrates its solutions to clients; and a café and a cafeteria-style restaurant with an outdoor patio. In addition, the 2800 and 2900 buildings had been redecorated to reflect the glass, metal, and wood design of the high-tech structure, whose design was recognized by the Kansas City chapter of the American Institute of Architects.[18] The new building's dramatic entryway immediately gives visitors a sense of the futuristic style that permeates the campus and artfully reflects the company's vision.

Further down Rockcreek Parkway, the development building had also been completed, providing 200,390 square feet of space for *Cerner*'s software development group.

At the dedication ceremony, *Cerner* President Trace Devanny followed up on the remarks about *Cerner*'s growth that Patterson had discussed at the groundbreaking two years earlier. In 2001, Patterson said that *Cerner* would one day be a multibillion-dollar company. At the dedication ceremony, Devanny stated that the company had earned $752 million in revenues the previous year and was on its way to becoming the billion-dollar company Patterson had foreseen.

Holden remarked that *Cerner* was part of Kansas City's strong base of technology and life sciences companies and lauded the company as "one of Missouri's fastest-growing companies and one of our state's largest employers."[19]

Going Public

By mid-1986, *Cerner* executives had become firmly convinced that healthcare IT was an enormous growth industry and that *Cerner* had built the foundation on which it could become a leader.

The next step in facilitating the company's growth was to go public, which would enable it to raise cash, simplify mergers and acquisitions, and implement a stock ownership plan. On October 24, 1986, *Cerner* filed for a proposed initial public offering (IPO), or first sale of stock. Illig stated that the offer was "the key to the company's financing for the long term."[20]

Elaborating on the reasons for going public, Illig said that "as a public company, we had more credibility.... The decision to be a public company was driven in part by the fact that it was a less expensive way to raise capital, and in part by the fact that we had a venture capital investor that expected the thing to be a public company at some point so that they would have the liquidity to move their investment through the investment cycle process and realize the return."[21]

He added that stock options were another "currency" that *Cerner* would be able to offer to its associates, the people who "came into this grand scheme with us and put their careers on the line to help make it successful." Stock options would help make associates "a part of the equation from an equity standpoint," Illig said, which fit into the company's culture of sharing the rewards.[22]

Even more important, however, was the impact that going public would make on the medical industry.

Illig said, "The real driver was our need to be more credible to the buyers—those people that were looking at us, wondering, knowing that the decisions that they were going to make were going to be decisions that would carry them across [many] years, that we were going to be around for the long haul."[23]

Cerner began the IPO process by hiring two investment banks, Alex Brown & Sons and Kidder, Peabody & Co., to lead the company through each step and help it acquire investors, or underwriters. The banks then filed a registration statement with the U.S. Securities and Exchange Commission (SEC), which contained information about the IPO, as well as company information such as financial statements, management profiles, and descriptions of how the money would be used.

The next step in the process was the SEC's "cooling off" period, in which the agency investigates all the information in the registration statement. During this period, *Cerner* executives and the two banks prepared an initial prospectus, also known as a "red herring," which included a complete overview of the company, including its goals and risks.

"You've got to come clean with all your financial information," said Illig, who led the *Cerner* team that wrote the prospectus. "You've got to be very exhaustive in your description of all the things that might go wrong in terms of the risk factors that are highlighted in that document."[24]

The risks section of the prospectus, titled "Certain Factors," included a segment about the company's dependence on hardware manufacturers: "*PathNet*® is designed to operate on computers manufactured by Digital Equipment Corporation (Digital) and Texas Instruments Corporation (TI). Any significant failure by Digital or TI to meet the company's hardware requirements would have a material adverse impact on the company's operations."[25]

Another risk factor included in the prospectus was "variations in revenues and earnings," primar-

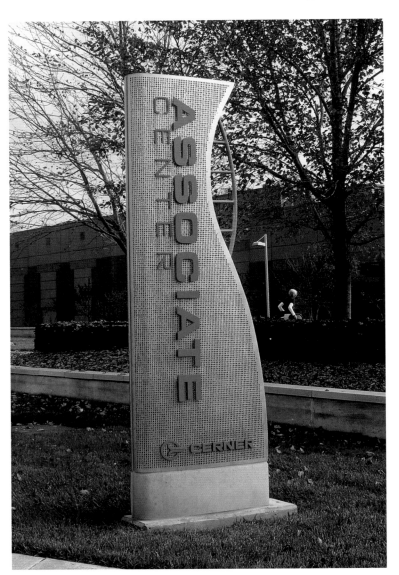

ily from the sale of *PathNet*®, "which has ranged from $100,000 to $3.3 million per installation."[26] Working on the red herring and all the other IPO materials was an all-consuming task for Illig and his team.

"It was kind of 'all hands on deck' from a *Cerner* standpoint," Illig said. "We did not have a large financial staff at that point. Maureen Evans, who was our controller and really our chief financial person in those days, put a lot of time into it. It was kind of a 20-hour-a-day effort for a period of a month or more to pull off the public offering."[27]

With the red herring in hand, *Cerner* executives and their bankers put on the obligatory "dog-and-pony" road show to court investors. They traveled to approximately 12 U.S. cities, as well as to London and Geneva.

Their presentations resulted in agreements with 59 underwriters, and on December 5, 1986, *Cerner* became a public company traded on the Nasdaq exchange with the ticker symbol CERN.[28] Originally priced at $16 a share, the 1 million shares offered raised $16 million.

A Quality-of-Life Campus

After buying Rockcreek Office Park in 1994, *Cerner* invested heavily in making the campus an attractive and desirable place to work. The Associate Center, built across the street from the 2800 building in 1995, was designed to enhance quality of life for associates and their families by providing childcare and exercise facilities.

Like other high-tech industries, the annual turnover rate at *Cerner* is high. In 1999, for example, the rate was 18 to 20 percent, in spite of 16,000 new applications and 900 new hires the previous year.

The company hoped the new benefits at the Associate Center—in addition to *Cerner*'s tradition of encouraging education and promotions, as well as incentives such as tuition reimbursement and

Cerner's Associate Center, which houses the Athletic Club and the *Cerner*Kids Learning Center, was designed to help the company stand out as a desirable place to work. (*Photo by Antonia Felix.*)

stock options—would help *Cerner* stand out from many other regional companies and persuade associates to build long-term careers with the company.

"We have an opportunity to attract top talent," then-Chief People Officer Stan Sword said in 2000. "In today's competitive job market, companies such as *Cerner* have to find unique ways to draw talented individuals."[29]

Retaining employees, and developing the company's knowledge base with those individuals who advanced through various teams, is a top priority supported by the extensive and non-traditional benefits that *Cerner* provides. One of the more unusual perks occurs at an associate's 10-year anniversary, at which time he or she is invited to dinner at Patterson's home.

The Associate Center houses the *Cerner* Athletic Club and *Cerner*Kids Learning Center. The fitness club, a state-of-the-art facility designed in the high-tech, ultramodern style of the rest of the campus, includes a conditioning room with treadmills and other equipment, an aquatics area, aerobics studio, basketball court, and racquetball courts.

CERNER DOCTRINE

ASSOCIATE SERVICES

CERNER'S APPROACH TO ASSOCIATE services is centered around an organization which supports the associates' day-to-day lives inside and outside of the working environment. It is a team collectively joined to support the associate by simply "making life easier."

This mantra is encapsulated by the services it provides, such as an orientation program, an on-site copy center, a day care, community outreach, and so on.

Together, the team performs precisely what its name implies, an emphasis and focus on services to benefit *Cerner*'s most valued asset— the associate.

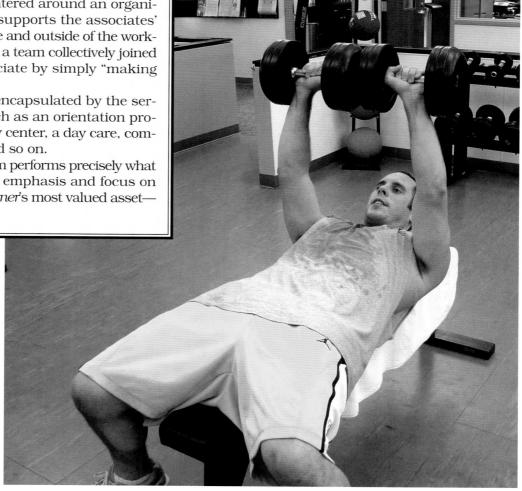

Software engineer Paul Perry works out in the conditioning room at the Athletic Club, the first of its kind in Kansas City. The fitness center also includes aquatics facilities, an aerobics studio, a basketball court, and racquetball courts. More than half of *Cerner*'s Kansas City associates are members of the club and pay only a low annual fee to use it. *(Photo by Antonia Felix.)*

When it opened, the on-site health club was the first of its kind in Kansas City.[30] Associates pay a low annual fee to use the club, and the company subsidizes most of the cost. In 2005,

The *Cerner*Kids Learning Center (below and insets) is an attractive option for associates with young children. Parents feel secure knowing their kids are close by, and the center's presence helps enhance the family–friendly atmosphere on campus. *(Photos by Antonia Felix.)*

more than half of *Cerner* associates who worked at the company's Kansas City headquarters were members, and on any given day, associates could be seen carrying gym bags to and from the center. For those living outside the Kansas City area, the company also reimburses part of the cost of associates' memberships at private health clubs.

*Cerner*Kids Learning Center, a Montessori-based program for children from ages 6 weeks to 6 years, is an enormously popular benefit for associates with families. Jan Gavin, who joined *Cerner* in

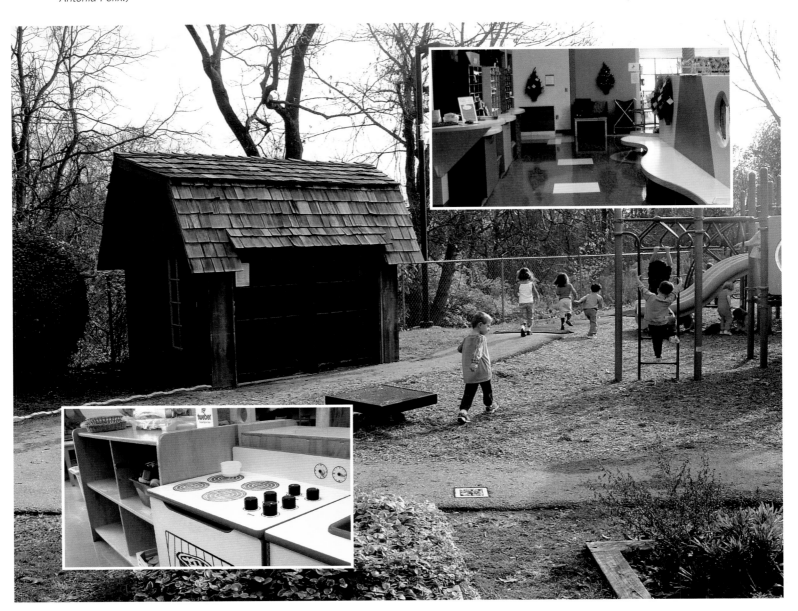

1985, remarked that having her children on campus made *Cerner* feel like a second home. "I feel I've grown up at *Cerner*," she said, "and now my kids are growing up there, too."[31]

When Stephanie Kobel interviewed for a job at *Cerner*, the *Cerner*Kids Learning Center clinched it for her. "When I heard they had the day-care center here, that's what sold me," she said. Stephanie and her husband, Rob, were comforted to know that their preschooler, Blake, was always just a building away.

"There's definitely a more positive attitude around here with programs like these," Rob Kobel said.[32]

For a feature story on *Cerner*'s family-friendly programs, Kansas City television station WDAF reported that "*Cerner* is a rare find. In fact, less than 10 companies in the greater Kansas City area have on-site day-care centers. Nationwide, the statistics aren't much better. [In a] survey of 1,000 companies, only 9 percent offer child care at or near the workplace, and fewer than 50 percent have formal policies on flex time."[33]

Offering a place to work out, swim, or practice yoga to relieve the stress of work was just one of the "Work/Life Balance" benefits developed at *Cerner*.

The family-oriented aspects of these initiatives are visible in the cafeteria, where a child can often be seen eating lunch with a parent, or in the fitness center, where couples play racquetball or work on training equipment together. In late October every year, families gather for a "Trunk or Treat" Halloween event in the parking lot; and on Friday nights, associates take advantage of Parent's Night Out, a program that offers Friday night child care at the Associate Center.

Other benefits designed to bring balance into associates' lives include private meditation rooms, new mother convenience rooms, an on-site ATM, postal services, a dry cleaner, and metro bus service to the campus with the Kansas City Area Transportation Authority. The company also provides regular health screenings and immunizations for associates and their children.

As one of the leading IT companies in the medical industry, *Cerner*'s long list of benefits is a strong draw for talent, as well as an expression of its overall commitment to health.

Combined, all of these benefits produced an atmosphere of high morale and job satisfaction at

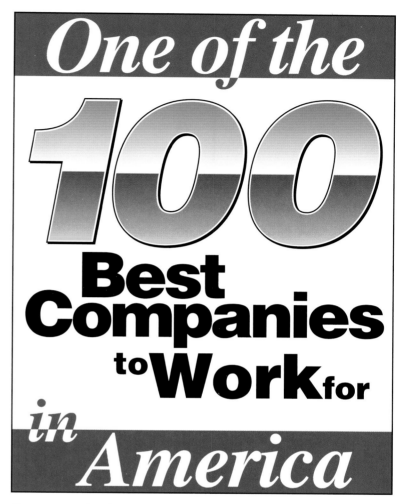

Cerner was nationally recognized in 1999 as a great place to work when it made *Fortune* magazine's list of the "100 Best Companies to Work for in America."

the company, which resulted in *Cerner* being named one of *Fortune* magazine's "100 Best Companies to Work for in America" in 1999. The companies who made the list were chosen on a point system based on a series of surveys, comments, and print and video materials supplied by about 1,000 companies under consideration that year.

Fortune's summary of *Cerner*'s work environment, which earned the company a place on the list, read: "Everything is up to date in Kansas City: on-site Montessori center, fitness center with swimming pool and basketball court; flexible work schedules; immunizations and health screenings for employees and dependents. *Cerner* supplies clinical information systems to health-care organizations. Employees seem ecstatic."[34]

Integrating life-balance programs and services into the work environment puts the philosophy of "treating others as you would like to be treated" into practice. The quality-of-life benefits at *Cerner* are another extension of a company culture that had always endorsed the "balance" of a work hard/play hard philosophy.

"I think one of the things that we've always felt is that it's not only important to work hard, but it's important to have a good time," Illig said. "Sometimes when we work so hard, we forget how important it is to have a good time, but there is a work hard/play hard part of the culture that has endured, and it's a very important part of what *Cerner* is."[35]

The "ecstatic" attitude observed by the *Fortune* list is backed up by Illig's view of *Cerner*'s positive and friendly atmosphere. "I think we enjoy each other's company," he said. "We enjoy the environment that we're working in. We enjoy the challenge that we're up against, and in that mode, [we] have bright, aggressive people. It's a lot of fun to do things when we're not necessarily working."[36]

The strong sense of community within the company has been borne out in the way associates pull together to help each other during difficult times.

"We all reach out to one another in a time of need," said Lupe Coursey, an associate whose 13-year position as administrative assistant earned her the unofficial title of "the voice of *Cerner*."[37] As an example of what she called the "extended family" feeling of the company, Coursey recalled Patterson's participation in a fundraiser in which associates pitched in to help a family. "We were having a drive for one of our associates who had a very sick husband at the time. One of the things that Neal had to do at the fundraiser was the Macarena in front of the associates. He was on his way to this fund drive, and he said, 'Lupe, teach me how to do the Macarena in five minutes!' So I stood up there and taught him how to do the Macarena."[38]

Cerner Virtual University

New solutions, new clients, and an expanding number of associates prompted *Cerner* to look for a new approach to training in the 1990s. The company's training model developed by Patterson and Campbell in 1996 had quickly evolved into a new organization within the company called *Cerner* Virtual University (CVU). A major aspect of training associates on *Cerner* solutions, their installation, and how to train clients to use those solutions, was the formation of a comprehensive, standard learning program that could be scaled to accommodate a variety of class sizes.

The company had taken its first step toward this goal in 1995 with the debut of the Associate Conference. That year, *Cerner* had 1,354 associates, a 24 percent increase from the year before. The conference provided the entire group with a full week of focused training, including hands-on demonstrations of solutions and skill development classes.[39]

The theme of *Cerner*'s new training philosophy involved shifting the idea that "knowledge is power" to "knowledge sharing is power." This was a dramatic change from the traditional business mindset in which highly skilled individuals feel empowered by holding specific pieces of knowledge in their field.

Among the systems for creating a fluid, communal knowledge system is My*Cerner*, an internal associate knowledge portal that began as an intranet program named Athena. The company also created a customized, personal portal for clients called the *Cerner* Knowledge Network (CKN). This portal gives clients a direct link to associates and to the information directly related to the *Cerner* solutions online at their facilities. My*Cerner*, CKN, and the company's Web site, cerner.com, have since been combined as a single point of reference in an effort called "fusion."

CVU designed its associate training around five learning principles: relevant learning, learning by doing, performance-based learning, just-in-time learning, and real-time learning.

"No amount of bells and whistles will save a training program if learners don't view it as relevant to what they do," Campbell said.[40] Consequently, *Cerner* Virtual University aligns its strategies with the annual goals of the company. It also maintains strong relationships with executives and senior managers who act as education sponsors for their areas of expertise. Programs are developed in direct response to *Cerner*'s business and client needs.

CERNER DOCTRINE

LEARNING AND KNOWLEDGE MANAGEMENT

*C*ERNER'S APPROACH TO LEARNING IS embodied in *Cerner* Virtual University's mission statement: To dramatically improve the human and organizational performance of *Cerner*'s associates, clients and business partners. *Cerner* strives to embody a culture of learning.

In the face of rapidly changing times, *Cerner* associates individually and collectively seek to continually improve their capabilities. The *Cerner* approach to learning allows associates to change and grow; it promotes *Cerner* as a learning organization capable of equipping the workforce of the future with the education and training they will need to succeed.

Cerner's approach to knowledge management creates the bridge from *Cerner*'s Intellectual Property to its associates and clients who apply the Intellectual Capital to their work.

The mantra for *Cerner* in this space is "What we learn today is used tomorrow." This means streamlining the creation and distribution of all intellectual capital and moving it very rapidly through both formal learning evens and knowledge access points (portals, communities, etc.) to the *Cerner* associates and clients who need it.

The synergies needed for success with this approach include:

- Alignment with the business
- Shared services infrastructure
- Transformation plan for learning
- Innovative delivery for the future
- Merging of learning, knowledge management, and performance support

---

"Learning by doing" is the most efficient way to teach associates about *Cerner* solutions, providing a hands-on, realistic setting in which to confront systems and situations as they arise.

Using the analogy of teaching a child how to ride a bike, Campbell said that the hands-on approach is the only way to go. "You put them on a bike, and you coach them and guide them and mentor them as they try to ride the bike. Installing software and designing software is very much the same way. You've got to get people on the bike. So we try to take that philosophy or approach in just about everything we do."[41]

The hands-on approach predominantly used at *Cerner* is called "goal-based scenario,"

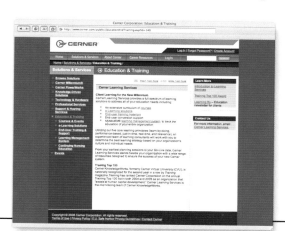

a simulation-based experience in which new associates are thrown into a real-life setting that they will one day encounter with clients.

"You simulate in compressed form what it's going to be like when they go out on the job and are working with clients," explained Campbell.[42]

With the help of *Cerner* mentors who are well-versed in the solution being learned and access to online information, associates learn how to use the resources at their disposal. Campbell explained:

Cerner Virtual University made *Training Magazine*'s Training Top 100 list in 2004 and 2005.

*If you encounter a situation, and you need infor-
mation, and you don't have it, who do you turn to?
How do you get the answers to those questions
quickly? Those are the metacognitive skills—or
learning-how-to-learn skills—that help you survive
if you're a Cerner associate. The reality is, our
business is complex enough that if you rely on formal training for every bit of technical knowledge
you need, you're never going to make it. But if you
can teach people how to learn, how to find the
answers or get up to speed quickly on their own,
then you've really enabled them to be successful.*[43]

Before the development of CVU, associates
were often forced to deal with *Cerner's* tough learning curve on their own. Matt Hodes, who came to
Cerner in 1988 as an installation consultant, recalled
the high anxiety of his first client site assignment. He
was sent to a client site to show them how to use
the 10 *PathNet®* lab applications they had purchased.
Armed with just a solutions manual, he imagined
that his clients would quickly discover that he had
had little exposure to the solutions.

"I was thinking that a client was going to stand
up in the middle of a session I was conducting and
say, 'You don't know what you're doing, do you?' "
Hodes said.[44]

Operating in survival mode, Hodes spent each
night in his hotel room learning what he had to
teach the client the next day. This went on for a full
week, and when he returned to *Cerner*, his boss
called him into his office.

Much to his surprise, Hodes' survival-mode
approach had worked. His boss told him that the
lab director had called to say that Hodes had done
a great job on the training trip. "That ... gave me the
courage to keep sticking my face into the middle of
something I didn't know and trying to figure it out
myself," he said.[45]

Associates are confident in their ability to meet
clients' needs due to CVU's third learning principle,
performance-based learning. Before meeting with
clients, associates are assessed on how well they
can put everything they have learned into practice.

"There needs to be an objective measure there
that says, 'Can they do it?' " said Campbell. "It's not
just, 'Can they throw back the knowledge that they
were presented in a class,' but can they actually do
it hands on?"[46]

With performance-based assessment, associates and their mentors are assured that clients
would receive top-notch service.

The fourth part of CVU's teaching strategy
is just-in-time learning. In client training, the
company discovered that when clinicians were
introduced to solutions too early, they would forget everything by the time the system was up and
running. Campbell explained this concept with
an example:

*I had one client who came to me and was so
pleased with herself because she had, with her
limited two classrooms, figured out how she
could get her 2,000 nurses and 500 doctors up to
speed, and she would only have to start training
on the application eight months before go-live.
I said, "Save your money. Don't do anything,
because anything that happens before ... three or
four weeks before go-live, is completely wasted.
They're not going to remember it." Learning
needs to happen just in time, right before you
need it.*[47]

Finally, the fifth tenet of CVU's philosophy is
real-time learning, which accounts for the fact
that the majority of learning occurs on the job.
After completing a curriculum about three or four
weeks before a new system is installed, clients
receive one-on-one, on-site coaching from a
Cerner associate.

"You've got *Cerner* associates that are working side by side with a client on the job, and they
provide the coaching and the consulting and the
guidance that support the formal training," said
Campbell. "That training again is very much learning by doing and performance-based. It's not sitting and listening to five days of lecture."[48]

The efficiency of client training programs at
Cerner Virtual University quickly translated into new
profits for the company. To everyone's surprise—
except Campbell's—CVU turned a profit after just
three years. Clients understood the value of investing
in training programs such as Web-based training
modules that simulate the solutions themselves,
and revenues from these programs made CVU a
self-sustaining segment of the company.

In addition to training associates how to present and install solutions, *Cerner* also developed a

program geared to associates whose jobs do not entail much client contact. This program, the Associate Client Experience (ACE), ensures that all associates understand how solutions are installed and serviced, and how the entire process is viewed from the client's perspective. For example, associates who develop software are able to visit client sites and support the conversion of new solutions.

CVU has become one of the top corporate training programs in the United States. In 2004, the program made its debut on *Training Magazine*'s Training Top 100 list, and ranked again in 2005. Rob Campbell, who attended the awards ceremony with Melanie Jescavage, manager of CVU's Learning Solutions Team, described what it takes to be named to the Top 100: "A number of criteria are reviewed, including the ability to measure the results of learning programs, the quality of those results, the innovation reflected in learning programs and solutions, overall investment per associate in time and dollars, etc. The bottom line is that it is very difficult to make the list."[49]

In addition to providing educational support for new associates, to enable familiarity with the company's IT solutions, *Cerner* also maintains an extensive internal IT system.

"Every company in the world has an internal IT organization," said Rich Miller, vice president of global resource information delivery. "The challenge here at *Cerner* is that it is an IT company. But we also have a need to have an internal IT organization to make sure that the way we use information technology is used in a very effective way. My focus today is to meet the needs of *Cerner*'s associates primarily and *Cerner*'s shareholders and to make sure the automation we need to execute our business is in place and operating well."[50]

Cerner's internal IT organization supports the infrastructure of devices necessary for associates to maintain their job productivity. This involves not only maintaining an extensive internal network, but also offering a round-the-clock Associate Response Center (ARC). Additionally, *Cerner*'s internal IT system provides comprehensive support to the complex solutions infrastructure. One example of this is its facilitation of *Cerner*'s Client Presentation environments, allowing presenters to most effectively demonstrate *Cerner*'s solutions.

In 1997 the complexity of *Cerner*'s ever-evolving solutions and the sheer volume of service requests from clients prompted a dramatic change within *Cerner*'s service and support system. The process was fine-tuned so that direct assistance and technical support would be immediately provided upon contact through the multiple channels in which clients can access *Cerner* for service.

"We wanted to attempt on first contact to connect clients with the individual capable of resolving the issue," recalled Miller.[51]

In 2004 the organization completed a massive conversion of *Cerner* Navigator, meeting an aggressive six month deadline. The undertaking increased the capabilities of *Cerner* Navigator, which tracks requests to fix issues, enhance, or add functionality to *Cerner* solutions. It also improved areas such as revenue predictability, access to information, individual accountability, and administrative operations.

Across the Country and Around the Globe

Sales of *Cerner*'s *PathNet*® solution boomed in the early 1990s, and by 1993, it had been implemented at 388 sites across the country. A highlight of 1993 was the conversion of *PathNet*® at Kaiser Permanente Northern California Region, which automated the laboratory system for approximately 3,500 physicians who provided care for nearly 2.5 million plan members. This installation made the California *PathNet*® site the largest community-based clinical information system in the world.[52]

With so many clients spread throughout the United States, *Cerner* made the decision to open several regional offices in 1993. The company hoped this strategy would help it maintain the long-term relationships it developed with each of its clients. These service-oriented relationships are reflected in the company's vocabulary.

"*Cerner* does not believe in forming typical vendor/customer relationships," stated the company's 1993 annual report. "A 'vendor' is someone who sells something to a 'customer.' Once the sale is complete, the so-called relationship is terminated. At *Cerner*, we form long-term relationships with

FIRST HAND FOUNDATION

IN 1995, *CERNER* CORPORATION and its associates founded the First Hand Foundation, a non-profit organization with a mission to directly impact the health status of young lives by providing needy children with healthcare services.

Through a committee comprised of healthcare professionals and *Cerner* executives, the charity reviews requests to help children who fall through the cracks of insurance coverage and state aid with specific medical expenses. *Cerner* matches associates' contributions dollar-for-dollar and ensures that all of the donations go directly to the children in need, instead of covering incidental expenses, such as administrative costs.

One case involved 7–year–old Jenna DePaul of North Kansas City, who was born with spina bifida. The girl needed a pair of $3,600 leg braces, but the DePauls' insurance would cover just $1,000 of the cost. The family earned too much to qualify for government assistance but could not afford to pay for the braces. The foundation stepped in with the needed $2,600.

The organization's other activities have included the funding of searches for bone marrow donors and organs for transplant surgeries, as well as cancer treatments and brain surgeries for children from foreign countries. In one case, the foundation provided prosthetics for a Pakistani girl who lost both legs and one arm to a land mine.[1]

Funding for the foundation comes primarily from *Cerner* associates, and the company matches each donation dollar for dollar. Associates donate through individual gifts and by organizing fundraising events. As a result of this generosity, First Hand has impacted more than 13,000 children in its first 10 years with grants totaling more than $4 million.

First Hand has many programs that allow associates to get involved and directly impact lives. Started in 2000, the *Love Bag*® Program, distributes bags to children entering the foster care system. Associates donate basic necessity and comfort items to fill these bags that help ease the stressful transitions faced by these children.

The R.E.A.c.C.H. Program offers associates the opportunity to provide clinical assistance to children around the world. Since 2001, R.E.A.c.C.H. (Associates Realizing Experiencing and Changing Children's Health) has hosted associates in countries in Romania, Peru, Brazil, and Jamaica.

For many Indian children suffering post-traumatic stress disorder (PTSD) from the 2004 Asian tsunami, help was granted thanks to the generosity of *Cerner* associates, First Hand, partner organizations, and numerous volunteers. Associates donated over $20,000 to create a

---

our clients to help them achieve their missions for clinical computing."[53]

More than a decade later, the company is still highly committed to developing its own version of the client relationship. "We are trying to redevelop what we call our client relationship model," said John Landis, vice president client operations, in late 2004. "We want to make sure that we are creating deep, valued, lasting relationships with our clients. This is

to really provide them with consultative expertise that will help them better understand how *Cerner* can improve their strategies as a health system and how we can couple health information technology with the core strategies of their organizations."[54]

One of the associates at the center of this improvement of client relationships is Jack Newman, Jr., executive vice president for strategic relationships. "In major metropolitan markets or for large project that uses eye movement desensitization and reprocessing (EMDR) for helping children psychologically devastated by the coastal attack.

The $1.1 million budget for 2005 allocates funds to the following programs that will directly impact the lives of more than 300 children and their families in 2005 alone:

- $766,000 for clinical services such as bone marrow transplants, physical therapy, and prescriptions.
- $219,000 for equipment such as prosthetics, as well as technologies that help kids acquire living skills and grow stronger.
- Nearly $88,000 for displacement or travel assistance for families who cannot afford travel to a specialized healthcare facility.
- $1,823 to help modify vans for children who require an accessible vehicle for their wheelchairs.
- $140,000 for non-traditional grants to provide a variety of services including *Love Bags*® for foster children, dental care for Spanish-speaking children, a leadership camp for 80 inner-city youth, and trips to countries all over the world for *Cerner* associates to bring medical care and knowledge to children in need.[2]

Following the catastrophic natural disaster of Hurricane Katrina on August 25, 2005, more than 1,000 associates came together to donate $150,977 to provide assistance to families evacuated to Children's Mercy Hospital in Kansas City. When Kashmir experienced a devastating earthquake several months later, a committee of Pakistani associates raised $13,275 toward the purchase of long-term temporary shelters, such as tents and tarps.

As co-founder of First Hand, Jeanne Patterson adds the role of philanthropist to the various positions she has held since being one of the first to join the company in 1981. In addition to her work for the foundation, Patterson serves on the Advisory Board of the Kauffman Foundation's Kauffman Scholars program and on the board of directors for the Ronald McDonald House Children's Charities in Kansas City.

In 2004, Patterson looked toward moving into a new form of public service by entering the race for the Fifth Congressional District seat in the U.S. House of Representatives. Even though she narrowly lost the election, it may not be her last. "She's looking to remain active in the political process in years to come," said her campaign spokeswoman, Cynthia Determan, after the election.[3]

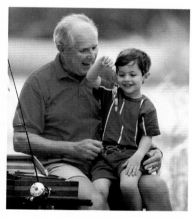

First Hand, a philanthropic, non-profit foundation established by *Cerner*, reaches out to thousands of children with medical needs whose families can not afford the necessary healthcare.

multistate systems ... I focus on proactively going out there, getting to know these people, and then entering into different sorts of arrangements than those you might traditionally enter. Oftentimes, they're risk/reward so the client can feel comfortable that we're not just selling them the software, but we ... stand behind it in terms of timely implementation [and] in terms of them getting measurable benefits out of it."[55]

Cerner's first branch offices were opened in Los Angeles, Dallas, Atlanta, Boston, and Washington, D.C., and in 1994, another branch was opened in Detroit. These offices enable associates to develop long-term relationships with clients.

During the 1980s and '90s, *Cerner* had also made great strides in expanding into the global marketplace, starting with the 1985 sale of *PathNet*® to four major hospitals in Canada's capital city,

Ottawa, Ontario. *Cerner* teams made the conversions at Ottawa General Hospital, Ottawa Civic Hospital, Riverside Hospital, and Queensway Carleton in 1986.

Although Canada technically marks *Cerner*'s international debut, the company usually refers to another contract as the starting point of its global sales. In June 1986, *Cerner* made a marketing agreement with McDonnell Douglas, granting it rights to market *Cerner* solutions under a private label in Europe.

Cerner expanded into the global marketplace with the 1985 sale of *PathNet®* to four major hospitals in Ottawa, Ontario, Canada. Soon after, an agreement with McDonnell Douglas brought *Cerner* solutions to Europe under a private label.

"By using McDonnell Douglas as our entrée into the international marketplace," said Patterson in 1988, "our advantage is an already established sales network through most of the English-speaking countries. Initially, and certainly over the next three years, our international focus is going to be on those countries."[56]

He also anticipated growth into other parts of the world. "In the long term, when we project three to five years, we also have an interest in the non-English-speaking countries."[57]

McDonnell Douglas paid $2 million for marketing rights, another $2 million for solutions and services, and $292,000 in royalties during 1986, the first year the contract was in effect.[58] The following year, *Cerner* earned royalties of $526,000 on the contract.[59]

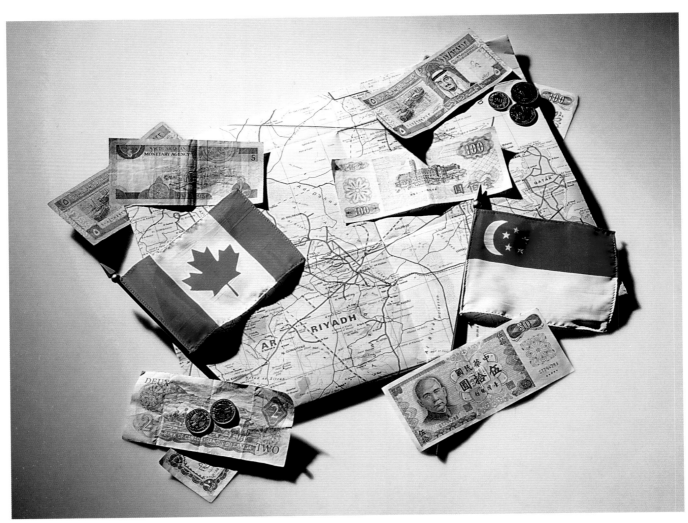

These international deals were just the beginning of *Cerner's* global identity. By 2004, the company would have clients in 12 foreign countries.

Acquisitions

During the 1990s, *Cerner* made several acquisitions to enhance the ongoing development of its *Health Network Architecture®* solutions. Each acquisition was made with the intent of increasing market share, acquiring specialized skill sets, or entering selective new markets. The first of these deals came in 1991 with the acquisition of Intellimetrics Instruments Corporation of Billerica, Massachusetts, and McDonnell Douglas Information Systems Ltd., in the United Kingdom.

Intellimetrics, which came to be known as *Cerner* East, was purchased to help develop *Cerner's* electronic medical record solution. In the McDonnell Douglas acquisition, *Cerner* assumed the private-label *PathNet®* contracts that McDonnell Douglas had made with the Northwest Thames Regional Health Authority, which implemented the solutions at 16 hospitals in England.

In 1993, *Cerner* acquired Megasource, Inc., to become the leader in the pharmacy information systems market. *Cerner's* pharmacy solution, *PharmNet®*, had been brought to market in 1989, and quickly became one of the most respected tools for that sector of healthcare. Along with *PathNet®*, the pharmacy solution was selected by Andersen Consulting's Hospital of the Future℠ as "representative of the healthcare industry's best clinical information system in its discipline."[60]

At the time of the acquisition, Megasource was the leading stand-alone pharmacy solution. *Cerner's* 54 *PharmNet®* clients combined with 319 Megasource MSMEDS clients to result in a new base of 373 *Cerner* Megasource clients. In this move, *Cerner* gained Megasource's accumulated, broad knowledge of pharmacy processes and its open systems interface engine called the Open Engine Application Gateway System.[61] This market-tested interface system fit in well with *Cerner's* vision of integrated solutions.

In 1998, *Cerner* acquired Multum Information Systems, Inc., for the purpose of embedding Multum content within Millennium. Multum, a Denver-based company, had created drug knowledge databases and had nearly completed a drug information software development kit (SDK) called *MediSource™* to be used in medical IT systems.

MediSource™ gives physicians, pharmacists, and other clinicians instant access to information about potentially harmful drug interactions, a comprehensive database of drug information, patient education materials, and other drug-related data. Medical IT solutions like *MediSource™* dramatically reduce adverse drug events, or ADEs, unwanted or harmful side effects as a result of a medication or a combination of medications. ADEs are the most common cause of unintentional injury or death in hospitals.[62]

"Multum's *MediSource™* solution is the only commercially available drug-dosing tool that supplies expert, person-specific clinical and drug utilization review data," stated *Cerner's* 1998 annual report.[63]

The same year as the Multum acquisition, *Cerner* entered into an agreement with General Electric (GE) Medical Systems to advance *Cerner's* radiology solution, the *RadNet®* Radiology Information System. *RadNet®* provides radiology departments with an efficient, computer-based alternative to manual, paper-based record-keeping systems. GE had developed an imaging technology called Picture Archive and Communication Systems (PACS), and together the two companies developed a solution that allows seamless access to both data and images.

In 1999, *Cerner* formed a strategic alliance with New Jersey-based Synetic, Inc., an e-commerce company. *Cerner* bought a 19.9 percent stake in Synetic's healthcare communications subsidiary, Synetic Healthcare Communications, Inc., (which, through a number of subsequent transactions, became WebMD Corporation) and developed a tool for providing clinicians with an Internet link to managed care plans, pharmacies, laboratories, and patients.[64]

The marriage of the two companies created "an entirely new form of communication between physicians and health plans," Patterson said after the announcement. "By providing physicians with online access to patient and plan-specific information, we can make healthcare services friendlier, less costly, and more responsive to physicians and patients alike."[65]

Cerner's acquisitions in the 1990s has actually helped to build on the company's vision of bringing fully integrated electronic solutions to medicine, as it continues to seek out partners that will help realize this mission.

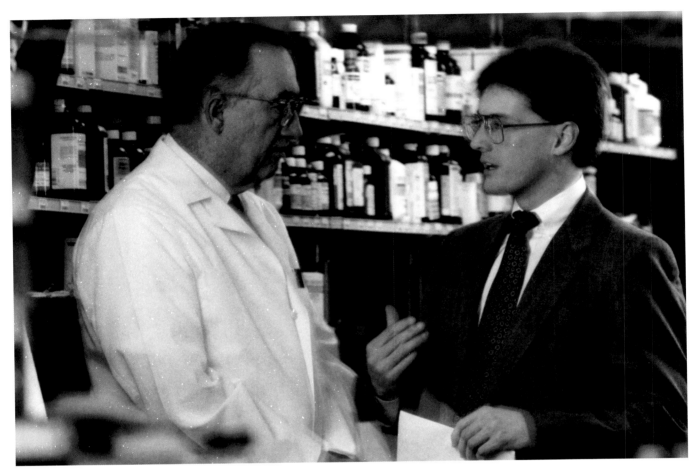

"While many of our competitors have a rollup mentality, in which they will simply acquire companies to cover the breadth of a new market segment, *Cerner* has had a core commitment to organic growth," said Jeff Townsend, chief of staff and executive vice president.[66]

Paul Black, *Cerner*'s chief operating officer and executive vice president, expounded by saying:

> Cerner *is more than simply catering to a financial plan, we are genuinely interested in improving and creating longstanding financial and clinical change that is going to benefit both clients and end-users.* Cerner *has consistently focused on the long-term, building from two concepts: the desire to automate a core clinical process and the recognition of requiring the necessary architecture to accomplish that. You can't create shortcuts to get to that final endgame, which is to provide a solution that will be broadly embraced and be broadly useful to a group of clinicians.*[67]

Cerner's *PharmNet®* solution debuted in 1989 and quickly became one of the leading tools for pharmacy automation. It was selected by Andersen Consulting's Hospital of the Future[sm] as "representative of the healthcare industry's best clinical information system in its discipline."

The company continued to acquire technology companies in the new millennium, including the May 2000 purchase of CITATION Computer Systems, Inc. Based in St. Louis, this company provided laboratory systems to about 300 small- to mid-sized hospitals in the United States, Canada, Latin America, and the Asia Pacific region. The transaction allowed *Cerner*'s newly acquired clients to "have unprecedented access to *Cerner*'s premier, integrated, enterprise-wide clinical systems," said Patterson.[68]

In November of that year, *Cerner* expanded its radiology solutions with the acquisition of

ADAC Health Care Information Systems. ADAC's technology, including a set of solutions called Envoi that utilized the imaging system *QuadRIS*, was integrated into *Cerner*'s Millennium radiology products.

"This acquisition broadens our market presence and enhances our knowledge capital in radiology," Patterson said. "These additional footprints within the radiology segment further *Cerner*'s mission to make healthcare smarter, safer and more efficient."[69]

Cerner made new laboratory and radiology inroads in December 2001 with the purchase of Dynamic Healthcare Technologies (DHT) headquartered in Lake Mary, Florida. The new organization, *Cerner* DHT, began delivering three new solutions: *CoPathPlus* anatomic pathology system, *RadPlus* radiology information system, and *Premier Series LIS* clinical laboratory system.

"The DHT transaction is consistent with our acquisition strategy of identifying companies with talented associates, attractive client demographics, and solution functionality that can be incorporated into Millennium," said Devanny. "We look forward to serving Dynamic's strong client base of more than 600 healthcare organizations and providing access to our industry-leading clinical and financial solutions."[70]

Zynx Health, Incorporated, a subsidiary of Cedars-Sinai Medical Center that provided knowledge and best practice solutions that were considered the industry standard, was acquired by *Cerner* in May 2002. *Cerner* integrated Zynx's evidence-based content into its Millennium knowledge solutions such as *Discern Expert*®, adding an extensive library of "rules" that informs and alerts clinicians of potential patient issues. Although *Cerner* divested Zynx in 2004, its portfolio of knowledge partners has continued to grow.

Other notable acquisitions in the early millennium included the purchase of Germany's Image Devices GmbH in August 2002 and the attainment of Beyond Now Technologies, Inc., based in Overland Park, Kansas, in September 2003.

In January 2005, *Cerner* expanded its physician practice solutions by acquiring the Medical Division of VitalWorks, Inc., a leader in the fast-growing private physician office information technology market. Approximately 100,000 physicians were already using *Cerner* solutions to manage their practices, and the VitalWorks acquisition brought the company an additional 30,000 private physician clients.

Patterson explained that this market addresses the national movement toward healthcare IT: "With Washington squarely focused on the physician practice space and with President Bush's call to action for each American to have a personal health record within 10 years, we believe there is a significant opportunity to make our vision of establishing a new medium between the physician and the person a vital reality," he said.[71]

The acquisition in May 2005 of Axya Systèmes, a Paris-based healthcare information technology company, further expanded *Cerner*'s international presence. Specializing in financial, administrative, and clinical solutions for hospitals, Axya has a diverse client base throughout France, Switzerland, and Morocco.

"*Cerner* and Axya have a shared mission to improve the quality of healthcare around the world," said Trace Devanny, *Cerner* president. "Together we are better positioned to capitalize on the many opportunities available in all segments of the French healthcare market. Axya is an excellent fit within *Cerner* because of our common cultures, complimentary solutions, and similar views on the importance of unified architecture."[72]

Each of the company's acquisitions has been integral to advancing the original vision of improving healthcare in the United States and throughout the world. As stated in the 2000 annual report: "We see a transformed healthcare system in the future, with healthcare organizations that make no avoidable errors, efficiently operate in a paperless environment, consistently deliver the highest quality of care based on the most current knowledge available, and are highly sensitive to the needs of the persons and communities they serve."[73]

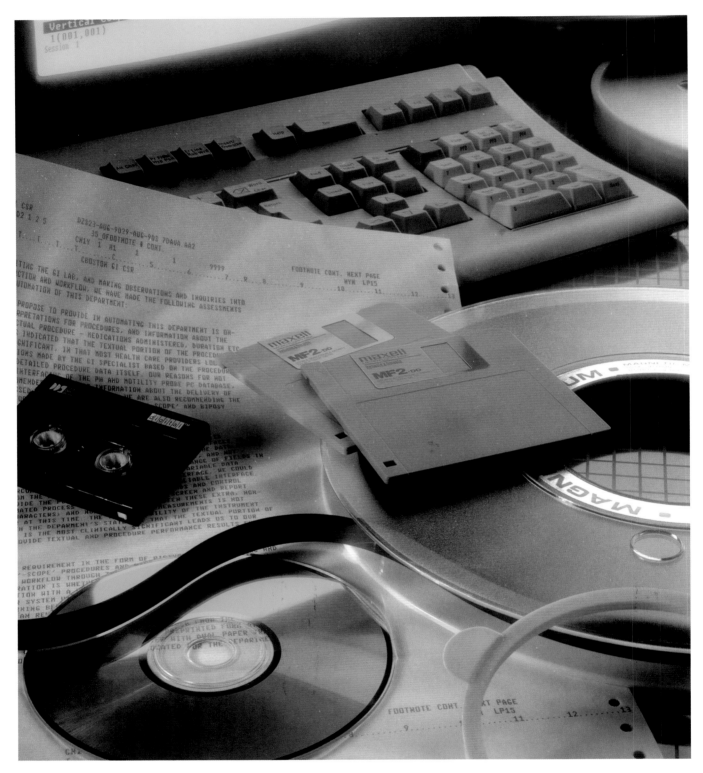

Each of *Cerner*'s solutions has emerged from the company's original concept of a unified architecture to automate healthcare processes. These systems include Clinical Solutions that enhance healthcare delivery, Direct Care Solutions that minimize errors and delays, Knowledge-Driven Care Solutions that put critical information at users' fingertips, Specialty Care Solutions that target specific areas of medicine, Consumer and Community Solutions that put the person at the center of health records, and Financial and Operational Solutions that help healthcare facilities conserve resources.

CHAPTER FIVE

TRANSFORMING HEALTHCARE: HOW *CERNER* SOLUTIONS WORK

Clinical discoveries or best practices published in a research paper are of little value unless the physician can use the knowledge easily and immediately when caring for patients. Cerner's goal is to close this information loop in healthcare—to increase the amount of new health information that can be incorporated into practice and to condense the amount of time it takes for the knowledge to reach physicians.

—Paul Gorup, *Cerner* co-founder[1]

FROM ITS FIRST LAB APPLIcation to an innovative Internetbased community healthcare connection to visionary plans for the next level of information technology, *Cerner*'s solutions have systematically changed the way medicine is practiced and enhance the healthcare system at every level.

Each of *Cerner*'s solutions has emerged from the company's original concept of a unified architecture that characterized its very first solution, *PathNet*®. As the founders and team of engineers became more familiar with healthcare delivery needs outside the laboratory, they strove to create solutions that would bring efficiency and cost-effective processes to virtually every area of medicine.

Clinical Solutions Enhance Healthcare Delivery

PathNet®'s successful debut in 1982 at St. John Medical Center in Tulsa gave the company a closeup look at hospital systems. During that first conversion they began discussing other clinical areas in which they could develop solutions based on the company's *Health Network Architecture*®. Illig had spent time talking to surgeons at St. John about their IT needs, and from these meetings emerged an idea for a surgical IT system. Although this solution would not appear on the market for several years, the seed was planted early in the company's history.

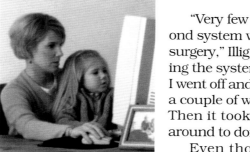

"Very few people know that the second system we actually [designed] was surgery," Illig said. "While we were turning the system on at St. John in Tulsa, I went off and talked to the surgeons for a couple of weeks to work on a design. Then it took us 10 more years to get around to doing [a] surgery [solution]."[2]

Even though surgery was on its map, the next *Cerner* solution to debut addressed the needs of pulmonary medicine. The first pulmonary information system, introduced in 1987, was the original solution in a new line called the *MedNet*® *Internal Medicine Information System.* Like the other clinical solutions that would follow, the pulmonary system automated several facets of the department including procedure requests; patient and therapist scheduling; and the processing, validation, and presentation of results. The solution also generated workload and billing reports, as well as summaries of clinical activities.

Pulmonary medicine shares many of the needs of the lab, but its specific requirements challenged engineers. "What was really hard was taking the

Cerner's person-centered healthcare philosophy entails community IT systems in which people actively participate in maintaining their electronic medical records and communicate with clinicians through e-mail and online chat rooms.

concept that we'd learned in a fairly narrow setting, the laboratory, and figuring out how to expand that into an architectural platform that we could use to do all these areas," Illig explained.[3] He and Patterson realized that although it would not exactly be simple to modify, their original architecture would support solutions for internal medicine, as well as other areas of care.

"You can't do anything in healthcare without information, and a lot of that information comes from the lab," Illig said. "So it's always been what Neal and I call the nexus of the information equation inside healthcare. But having done it and done all the departments of it around the *PathNet®* system, we really learned to appreciate that the architecture that we had developed could be not easily, but readily, transferred to the other areas inside healthcare."[4]

In 1988, *Cerner* turned to radiology for its next solution in the *MedNet®* line. The *RadNet® Radiology Information System* brought automation to diagnostic radiation and radiation oncology departments and efficiency to their operational and management needs. Replacing paper-based systems with an electronic, computer-based system, *RadNet®* was designed to schedule appointments, modify orders, track patients in the hospital or clinic, locate films, transcribe reports, and issue productivity reports.

"We are exceptionally pleased with the preliminary feedback and are confident that *RadNet®* will set new standards in clinical computing for diagnostic and therapeutic radiology," the company's annual report stated the following year.[5]

Cerner later enhanced its radiology solution when it did some joint development work with General Electric to expand upon GE's imaging product in 1998. Picture Archiving and Communication Systems (PACS) were a new addition to the field of medical IT that converted X-ray films to digital data that could be accessed on a computer screen. Not only did PACS allow instant, easy access to X-rays by any number of clinicians at the same time, they eliminated the need to retake X-rays by keeping a database of images for each patient.[6]

In 2000, *Cerner* released the *ProVision™ PACS Workstation*—available as an enhancement of *RadNet®* or as a stand-alone solution—to provide access to digital radiology images with a simple-to-use interface. This "real-time radiology" solution decreased the turnaround time for reports from

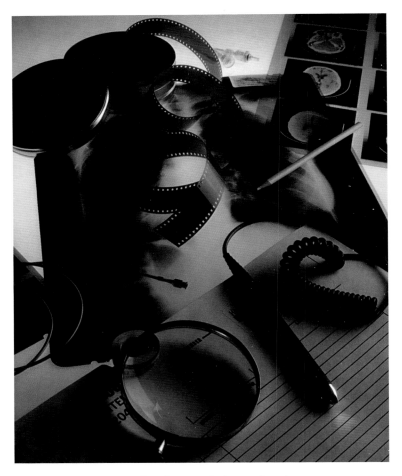

RadNet® was one of the first *Cerner* solutions to target an area outside of the hospital laboratory. The system helps automate radiology department procedures such as scheduling appointments, modifying orders, tracking patients, locating films, transcribing reports, and issuing productivity reports.

hours or days to just minutes by providing instant access to digital images on the computer and creating an automatic storage system. The solution also included an optional 3-D feature.

All Children's Hospital of St. Petersburg, Florida, provided a prime example of the far-reaching benefits of these solutions. The hospital had committed to becoming a paperless, streamlined medical facility, and its use of *RadNet®* and *ProVision™ PACS* helped the hospital reach its goal.

Cerner included this success in its marketing materials, saying, "the organization has reduced the need for film filing and retrieval, decreased reporting turnaround times, and provided instantaneous image availability. By eliminating unread imaging studies, All Children's has also eliminated lost films and lost revenue, minimized dictation errors, and improved outcomes."[7]

The *MedNet®* family of solutions continued to expand with the development of a pharmacy solution in 1989. The *PharmNet®* pharmacy system allowed clinical pharmacies—both inpatient and outpatient—to make a quantum leap forward in efficiency and accuracy. Designed to put all types of pharmaceutical orders on one screen, this solution streamlines orders for medication and automatically maintains patient profiles and pharmaceutical inventories.

With *PharmNet®*, a pharmacist can check orders for possible interactions with other medications and foods, as well as duplicate therapies, and easily obtain information about recommended dosages for particular medical conditions. The pharmacist and other clinicians can type in notes that are sent instantly to other clinicians for comment or follow-up. *PharmNet®* also provides medication administration records automatically or on demand, and automatically captures charges.

General Hospital (Grey Nuns) of Edmonton, Alberta, Canada, converted to all of *Cerner's* available solutions in the late 1980s, after administrators discovered that other IT companies could not deliver the integrated system they needed to allow communication between several departments and clinicians.

According to hospital President and CEO David Hart, *Cerner* also stood out from the competition with its seamless approach to integrating its solutions with the hospital's current systems. He said, "Other software companies seem to say, 'Here's our system and the way we have addressed your needs. Now develop your data and the way you provide care around it.' *Cerner*, on the other hand, allows our care providers to mold the system to their current operations."

Hart believed that *Cerner* had become the leader in the industry because it had the most far-reaching vision. "*Cerner* has some of the brightest talent in the industry dedicated to technology," he said. "The senior management understands the industry of information technology and is able to stay ahead of how that technology affects healthcare providers."[8]

MedNet®, *Cerner's* first foray out of the laboratory, was just the first destination on the company's long-term roadmap. The founders had boundless confidence in their architecture's flexibility and its ability to meet the needs of many clinical departments. It would not be an easy task, but they knew their vision of improving healthcare through IT was realistic. As former Andersen Consulting executives, Patterson, Illig, and Gorup were also accustomed to setting aggressive goals and timetables for software solutions across a wide variety of industries, and this experience helped formulate their expectations for *Cerner*.

"We went in with one design, but that design expanded over time," Illig recalled. "We had made commitments on when we'd have things up and running, but this was all stuff we had done many, many times before at Andersen, which was to take a design and convert it to something that worked and turn it on." Although medical IT was a new industry for the

CERNER DOCTRINE
LEADERSHIP

THE POWER OF AN ORGANIZATION lies in its ability to combine the talents and dreams of many individuals, all contributing to a common vision and strategy, with a goal of providing outstanding benefits for the clients it serves. *Cerner's* leadership combines the strength of dedicated, long-tenured executives who shaped the corporation with the fresh insights of less-tenured but talented individuals who offer their expertise in technology and the industry.

Together, they lead the organization with a combination of vision, experience, perseverance, flexibility, commitment, and dependability, a combination that allows *Cerner* to meet the dynamic needs of the healthcare industry. The company succeeds by combining its internal leadership with the valuable input it receives from its clients.[1]

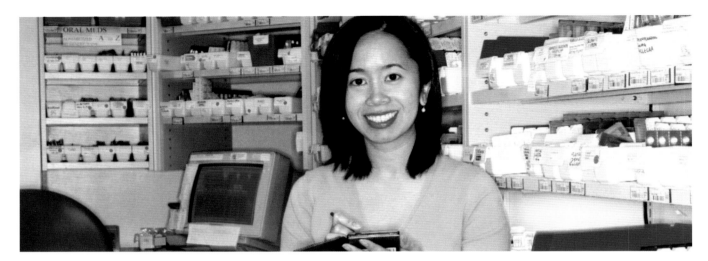

founders, they believed in their people, their ideas, and their vision. "The doability of it was really never in question," Illig said. "I think there were other people that probably would question it, but we never really did."[9]

Cerner's executives also realized that making mistakes had much more serious consequences in the healthcare industry than in the others with which they were familiar. Illig recalled that this reality became clear during the first *PathNet* conversions in the early 1980s. As he and Patterson talked about their lab solution while walking the halls of St. John in Tulsa, they reflected on the impact of their work.

"This is really, really hard stuff because you're playing with people's lives," Illig said. "It's not like if you screw up in a manufacturing system, some part doesn't work where it's supposed to, and it slows up some order. This stuff, if you screw it up, if somebody's results get scrambled, that's serious stuff."[10]

During the development phase for *MedNet* solutions, Patterson made it clear that *Cerner*'s method of expanding its solution line was very different than that of the competition. "We do see what we call 'natural bridges' into other clinical areas," he told *Healthcare Computing & Communication* in 1987. "Unlike the broad product line suppliers, however, *Cerner* is not following a strategy that attempts to 'piece' dissimilar products together. We believe that the healthcare industry of the future will demand systems built on a common architecture, with an emphasis on 'critical mission' systems that contribute to a comprehensive clinical database."[11]

PharmNet allows pharmacists to check orders for possible interactions with other medications and foods, as well as duplicate therapies, and easily obtain recommended dosage levels for specific medical conditions.

Computer hardware at the time these early solutions were being developed posed challenges, too. "This was an online, real-time system that was interacting with medical instruments and a big hospital computer that was sending information over to us," Illig said. "This was complex, real-time computing, and the computers were not nearly as stout as they are today. So we had lots of challenges, not only making the things work functionally but making them perform adequately."[12]

By 1990, *Cerner*'s solutions had reshaped the medical IT industry by offering system integration throughout the hospital. That year, *Cerner* solutions represented "the broadest integrated clinical information system in the industry," according to its annual report.[13]

Direct Care Solutions Minimize Errors and Delays

By 1991, more than 350 medical facilities across North America had implemented *Cerner* solutions. That year alone, the company sold 69 new *PathNet* solutions. By that time, 20 sites had converted to *RadNet* and another 20 had implemented *PharmNet*. Financially, it was a record-setting year for the company, which posted a 35 percent increase in revenues from the previous year to $77.2 million.[14]

In this exciting atmosphere of growth, the company got a jump-start on aggressive development of its electronic medical record (EMR) solution, which it named the *Open Clinical Foundation* (OCF), when it acquired Intellimetrics and hired Dr. David M. Margulies, a Harvard Medical School graduate and former chief information officer at Boston Children's Hospital, to direct development of the OCF.

The electronic medical record had been the subject of extensive research and debate for more than two decades, and it promised many benefits to the healthcare industry. First, a digital record could store data in a small space, in contrast to the bulky file rooms at most hospitals and doctors' offices. Also, the EMR would make patient information available to many people at the same time. Thirdly, information could be retrieved instantly, at the push of a button. This would allow physicians to free themselves from the time-consuming task of retrieving data from a paper record to spend more time with their patients.

One study, published in 1998, reported that the average hospital had approximately 17 separate records for each patient scattered throughout various departments.[15] An EMR would eliminate this redundancy. In addition, the EMR could be programmed to provide clinical alerts and flags to information from various departments, from the lab to radiology.[16] From the patient's perspective, the EMR would eliminate the need to provide a medical history at each stage of treatment, a system that relied primarily on a patient's imperfect memory.

In spite of these advantages, the EMR had been slow to catch on. One of the primary drawbacks was the issue of privacy and security. Records formatted for cyberspace were vulnerable to hackers and others who can determine how to sidestep passwords and other security measures. In spite of highly reliable encryption software, many people remained suspicious about EMR safety, and the fast-paced growth of technology had raised concerns about an erosion of attention to patient confidentiality.

"The unprecedented capacity of digital technology to acquire, merge, and disseminate data instantaneously encourages euphoria about the benefits of the technology, cynicism about the relevance of traditional privacy and confidentiality values, and fatalism about the future of privacy and confidentiality," warned one industry report in 2000.[17]

Additional concerns about the EMR that have been voiced over the years included high start-up costs, steep learning curves, and the question of whether doctors and other practitioners would be willing to enter data. But as early as 1991, *Cerner* firmly believed that the EMR would one day be the standard patient record. Giving credibility to that view, several bodies within the United States government began expressing interest in the possibilities of EMRs increasing efficiency and reducing healthcare costs.

In his 2004 State of the Union address, President George W. Bush highlighted the importance of moving toward wide acceptance of the EMR. "Our nation's healthcare system, like our economy, is also in a time of change," Bush said. "Amazing medical technologies are improving and saving lives. ... By computerizing health records, we can avoid dangerous medical mistakes, reduce costs, and improve care."[18]

A few months later, the president was more specific about the goals of his administration and the benefits of the EMR. "Within 10 years, we want most Americans to have electronic healthcare records," he told an audience at the Vanderbilt University Medical Center. "You not only save money, you improve the quality of care through the spread of good information. It lets these docs do their jobs; it eases the minds of the patients."[19]

Cerner's OCF solution was designed to address these issues. It records and archives vital patient information in a central repository, thus forming the foundation for electronic medical records. The OCF enabled the creation of a convenient, online patient chart that incorporates the management of medical documents, as well as voice, image, and interpretive data.

One of the greatest challenges of creating the OCF database was the lack of a standard terminology for all the terms used in healthcare, a field more vast and complex than banking, manufacturing, and other industries that had created a standard nomenclature when they developed IT systems.

"There are easily upwards of a million unique concepts in medicine, and it's a big job to go and give a name to all those things and assign a standard number," explained David McCallie, *Cerner*'s vice president of Medical Informatics and chief scientist.[20]

A PERSON-CENTERED PHILOSOPHY

CERNER CEO NEAL PATTERSON'S vision of healthcare IT entails a focus on the "person" rather than the "patient." This idea views healthcare from a lifetime perspective, in which a cradle-to-grave database of medical information exists for each person. Patterson began using this new terminology in the 1990s as a way of shifting the healthcare IT mindset from a collection of fragmented parts to a system focused on one basic element—the individual. He said:

Early in this, we saw that [healthcare] will continually evolve, but it starts and stops with the same thing. In the '80s, I did [use the term] patient as the noun, but in the '90s I stopped doing that, and I used the word patient as a modifier to the noun. The noun is the person. There is a kind of epiphany, if you will, of how simple it is and yet

how complex. The Mayo Brothers in Minnesota in the early 1900s, for example, created a group practice that basically said, "we'll work as a team for the purpose of helping a person."

But by far the majority of our delivery system is otherwise. There are all these fragmented pieces. Knowledge is so vast. [We], as a species, and the conditions that we get—there's so much to know, it has to be broken into specialties because it's just too big. It's broken into these specialties and sub-specialties, and no one had designed anything that coordinates it, connects it.[1]

Patterson's person-centered philosophy was part of the motivation for developing an entirely new type of *Cerner* architecture, HNA *Millennium*®, in the 1990s.

In an effort to promote the development of medical IT, the National Library of Medicine (NLM) took on the challenge of building a common language with a research project called Unified Medical Language Systems (UMLS). McCallie, who joined *Cerner* in 1991, incorporated elements of this project into the OCF, thereby creating one of the world's first commercial applications of UMLS.

"The problem was that NLM didn't intend for UMLS to become the national standard vocabulary because they knew that they really weren't staffed to maintain it and make it an official vocabulary," McCallie said. "They weren't in that business in a sense, but it was the closest thing that anybody had to something that could serve as a substitute for a standard vocabulary."[21]

McCallie explained that a national standard called the Systemized Nomenclature of Medicine (SNOMED), which had gone through various stages of development since the 1960s, had finally been expanded for broad use in medicine by 2003–04.

"The SNOMED model was derived in part from that UMLS work," he said, "so the work that I had done to create the UMLS infrastructure inside *Millennium*™ was reasonably adaptable to SNOMED, although they did have to make some changes."[22]

Cerner's EMR, called the *PowerChart*® *Electronic Medical Record System*, is an enterprise-wide solution that utilizes the patient information that was stored in the OCF. *PowerChart*® allows doctors to view, order, document, and manage the delivery of care from a PC workstation. Healthcare providers can browse through electronic pages as they would a paper record, instantly accessing information from every department in which the patient has received services.

The solution was designed to allow easy access to specific information through a table of contents and a search engine, which can be used to locate particular terms throughout the text. Freed from searching through the hospital for paper records, clinicians receive instant access to a patient's lab

results, emergency room records, radiology reports, and other information. They are able to make better informed clinical decisions by having a complete patient history and test results at their fingertips.

The second solution in the OCF family was *PowerOrders®*, *Cerner*'s version of Computerized Physician Order Entry (CPOE), a medical IT term defined as "a computer application that accepts the physician's orders for diagnostic and treatment services electronically instead of the physician recording them on an order sheet or prescription pad."[23]

One key goal of the CPOE is to reduce medication errors—the largest single cause of medical errors in hospitals—by substituting a doctor's handwriting with electronic data. *PowerOrders®* reduces the longstanding problem of other healthcare providers having to call the prescribing physician to clarify orders and enhances workflow throughout the hospital by automatically alerting the appropriate clinicians and departments to a patient's needs. This solution contains built-in order sets, which allow a physician to move swiftly through the ordering process in even the most complex cases, and access up-to-date information about a patient's condition.

PowerOrders® enhances patient safety with alerts and reminders about drug-food interactions and other precautions. These built-in tools help reduce another common healthcare problem, adverse drug events (ADEs), and provide information about medications involved in complex dosing orders, including automatic calculations of preferred

formulas. *Cerner*'s CPOE ensures that orders are not misplaced or misread and that patients are billed correctly. In addition, *PowerOrders®* was enhanced with a knowledge database that gives physicians instant access to the latest scientific and medical research to help them better treat each patient.

The University of Illinois Medical Center, a major teaching hospital with an average of 1,600 system users a day, provided an example of the dramatic impact that these two enterprise-wide solutions can have on a facility. After implementing *PowerOrders®* and *PowerChart®*, the hospital found that physicians spent 30 percent less time looking for charts, the number of patients seen without a medical record was reduced by 40 percent, physicians spent five fewer hours a week reviewing orders from residents, and *PowerChart®* saved $1.3 million worth of clinicians' time spent performing manual documentation tasks.[24]

The Nemours/Alfred I. duPont Hospital for Children was just one hospital in which Cerner's

Cerner's Community Health Model illustrates the company's vision of an automated system that enables physicians to make the best possible treatment decisions; gives people the resources to better manage their own care; and organizes medical data to help speed scientific discovery, improving the quality and delivery of healthcare.

CONNECT THE PERSON (2) BY PROVIDING A VIRTUAL PERSONAL HEALTH SYSTEM

STRUCTURE, STORE & STUDY THE EVIDENCE (3) TO CREATE NEW KNOWLEDGE

AUTOMATE THE CARE PROCESS (1) AND ELIMINATE THE PAPER

CLOSE THE LOOP (4) BY IMPLEMENTING KNOWLEDGE-DRIVEN CARE

CPOE solution has been put to the test. In December 2005, the Nemours/Alfred I. duPont Hospital for Children reported that it had substantially reduced medication errors through the use of *Cerner* Millennium solutions.

"We have demonstrated what comprehensive studies have shown: CPOE reduces the risk of medication errors, therefore improving patient safety and decreasing the rates of mortality," said Dr. Terri Steinberg, clinical applications manager at Nemours. "Nearly 100 percent of the 50,000 orders placed here each month by physicians and clinicians are automated and online, providing a closed loop of care for medication administration."[25]

In unifying the medication management process, Nemours' medication error dropped to nearly 70 percent less than hospitals that were not utilizing CPOE, according to the *Journal of the American Medical Association*. The number of medication errors also remained well below the national average. The 180-bed children's hospital supports more than 4,000 registered clinicians and was ranked one of the "Best Places to Work in IT" in 2005 by *ComputerWorld*.

"The successful and consistent use of CPOE at Nemours/Alfred I. duPont Hospital for Children sends a clear message to the marketplace that patient safety and CPOE are inexplicably connected," said *Cerner* President Trace Devanny.[26]

The Children's Hospital and Regional Medical Center in Seattle, which is consistently ranked by *U.S. News & World Report* and *Child* magazines as one of the best children's hospitals in the country, was another facility to realize the positive impact of CPOE. The hospital experienced a reduction in acute-care medication delivery time by 70 percent, as well as a reduced order-entry time from physician order to pharmacy execution by more than 70 percent.

"Our CPOE implementation was part of a major safety initiative in our hospital," said Dr. Mark Del Beccaro, clinical director of information services and associate chief of emergency medicine at Children's. "CPOE has helped our hospital maintain its high standard and … ensure that we keep our children safe and provide them with the best care available."[27]

By the end of 2003, the company had made "significant progress at implementing CPOE at a large number of client sites," according to the annual report, and *Cerner*'s CPOE was the solution "generating the highest level of industry attention."[28] That year, two medical consulting firms issued reports that recognized *Cerner*'s leadership in the CPOE field.

In its annual "Medication Safety Tools" report, Five Rights Consulting, Inc., awarded *Cerner* the best scores in "high priority" criteria among other solutions generally available in the marketplace. The report also described *Cerner*'s CPOE as "an elegant solution that will likely be an immediate hit with clinical staff." KLAS, another healthcare IT consulting company, confirmed *Cerner*'s top standing in its 2003 "CPOE Perception" report. *Cerner*'s CPOE was rated "above average" in nine out of 10 performance categories such as architecture, physician use, end-user presentation, and clinical decision support.[29] The following year when KLAS polled decision-makers of acute care provider organizations, an impressive 64 percent stated that they would look to *Cerner* when evaluating CPOE solutions.[30]

PowerOrders®, *Cerner*'s version of the Computerized Physician Order Entry (CPOE) system, ensures that doctors' orders are not misplaced or misread, and that patients are billed correctly.

Cerner also introduced a solution for nurses that automated and streamlined many acute care tasks. The *CareNet*® Acute Care Management System put all patient information in an easy-to-navigate view for nurses and other care providers across the hospital system. Nurses throughout the hospital can communicate in real time, see a list of patients they were responsible for, view orders for each patient, and update a patient's care plan.

In addition, knowledge embedded in the system prompts important alerts and protocols. For example, when a nurse inserts information about a patient who is at risk of experiencing a fall, the solution triggers a protocol to minimize falling and resulting injuries. At Our Lady of the Lake Regional Medical Center in Louisiana, the rate of patient falls was reduced by nearly 20 percent after the facility converted to the *CareNet*® solution.[31]

Another solution designed to streamline nurses' delivery of care, *PowerPOC*™, is a point-of-care system that focuses on administering medication and other bedside activities. Set up in mobile or stationary carts in the patient's room or on a handheld device, the solution includes bar-code verification of the patient's five "rights" of medication use: right patient, right medication, right dose, right route, right time. The five rights are a traditional part of medication safety that every nurse learns in nursing school, and this automated system helps ensure that these criteria for dispensing medication are met.

Charlotte Weaver, *Cerner* vice president and chief nurse officer of patient care, has received extremely positive feedback about the company's nursing solutions:

> They absolutely love it. We keep them linked into the patient's electronic record at all times so they can see what's new on their patient's chart, quickly see what those results are and the new orders, and come right back out to [the screen] where they were doing their work. It always keeps reminders in front of them, and the system through its clinical decision-support engine can ... trigger a best-practice guideline to prevent the most common kinds of problems that occur in acute-care organizations. These problems include falls risk, best practice for management of pain, wrong-side surgery prevention, follow-up on a need for restraints, the kinds of regulatory things you need to do to stay in compliance

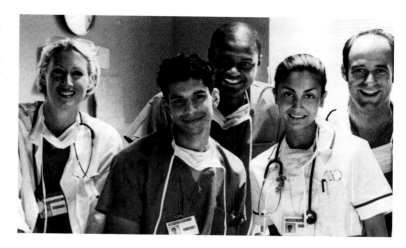

After *PathNet*®'s successful debut in 1982, *Cerner*'s founders utilized their experience in solving inventory problems for other industries to design an IT solution that would help automate surgical departments. However, *SurgiNet*® did not appear on the market until a decade later.

> with best practice around use of restraints. All those automatically happen.
>
> The other part that takes work off of nurses' shoulders is that the system can send requests for materials and for referrals to other members of the care team. Before, nurses would have to manually fill out those requisitions, pick up the phone, place an order, write out an order, and now the system can do all that. So what we hear from nurses is, "This takes work away; I can't imagine working without it."[32]

Cerner's *SurgiNet*® Perioperative Solutions was based on the design that Patterson and Illig had discussed 10 years previously during the first *PathNet*® conversion. Perioperative, or "around the time of surgery" tasks that were automated in this system include the coordination of staff, materials, equipment, locations, and patients. The solution alerts caregivers when supplies are about to expire, improving safety and providing for better inventory management. Culled from the founders' previous experience in solving inventory problems for clients at Andersen, this feature was a striking new development in medical IT.

"For the first time in healthcare, we are able to apply some of the same good management practices around inventory turn and control that are applied to other industries," said Pat Modlin, director of engineering at *Cerner*. "We provide a solution that brings together the clinical needs of surgical care with management of the inventory to create the best outcome for both patient safety and the financial viability of the organization."[33]

SurgiNet® also automated the billing process of surgical care. "Before we implemented *SurgiNet®*, we had three full-time employees doing charges manually," said Oscar Lamas, clinical supervisor at Torrance Memorial Medical Center in California, a facility with 15 operating rooms that conducts 17,000 procedures a year. "Now we have our nurses documenting, and charges are sent immediately to our charge services during the process. As a result, we have eliminated late charges, and our per-case revenues increased 17 percent over the past year (2003)."[34]

As the number of people using hospital emergency rooms soared, emergency medicine had also become increasingly complex. From 1992 to 2002, ER visits rose from 89.8 million to 100.2 million visits a year, an increase of 23 percent. At the same time, approximately 15 percent of the ERs in hospitals across the country closed.[35] All told, emergency room visits account for approximately 40 percent of all hospital admissions, making this a highly overcrowded area of care.

To address these unique challenges, *Cerner* developed the *FirstNet® Emergency Medicine Information System*, which focuses on improving patient safety as well as the bottom line. This solution includes a system for faster patient registration, a complaint-specific physician documentation system tailored to the ER, an electronic medical record, a coding system to facilitate billing, risk management tools with drug interaction alerts, and printouts that provide people being discharged with information about prescriptions and instructions for follow-up care.

The solution also includes an electronic triage form that automates the documentation performed by the nursing staff upon each person's arrival.

Cerner expanded the market for its Direct Care solutions by tailoring them to work for smaller organizations, including physicians' offices, clinics, and group practices. The *PowerChart Office® Management System*, which includes an EMR, was designed to provide these organizations with an increased level of efficiency, improved communication with an Online Patient Support component, and instant access to patient information. Just as the company's larger systems increase efficiency and enhance communication in a hospital setting, *PowerChart Office®* scaled the solutions to venues that serve smaller populations.

In 2001, Dr. Anthony Alfieri began using the solution to automate the practice of his 17-physician group, Delaware Cardiovascular Associates. Since the solution was implemented, the practice had experienced a $1.98 million return on its investment by 2004 due to the solution's automated coding process for billing, the reduction of no-shows for appointments, and the elimination of dictation services.

Rather than dictating a medical visit that would be sent to a transcriptionist, the *PowerNote®* module of *PowerChart Office®* allows the doctor to log the visit through a series of specialized templates, which automatically creates an electronic record of the visit. All of this is done in the same amount of time it would take to do traditional dictation, but the solution cuts out the traditional next step of transcription. Alfieri also observed that the presence of the system draws a very positive reaction from his patients.

"Patients want to see a physician who uses the computer; they realize it improves quality of care," he said. "Consequently, there has been robust patient enthusiasm for this system."[36] Alfieri added that the

Individual physicians' offices, clinics, and group practices are also able to take advantage of healthcare IT with *Cerner* solutions such as the *PowerChart Office Management System®*.

solution provides clear, comprehensive materials for patients to take home that help them coordinate their follow-up needs.

"When every patient is done seeing their physician, they receive a summary sheet, which is a typewritten page with the patient's medicines, allergies, problems, and procedures," he said. "Additionally, when a new medicine is prescribed, the patient receives a three-page information sheet about the medicine."[37]

Knowledge-Driven Care
Puts Information at Clients' Fingertips

When *Cerner* introduced its first Knowledge-Driven Care solution in 1990, "decision support," was a buzzword in the medical IT industry, but physicians remained skeptical about computer-assisted decision-making.

Among a few other decision support systems on the market, one well-known product, DXplain, had been developed at Massachusetts General Hospital by medical IT pioneer G. Octo Barnett, M.D. DXplain was designed to formulate input about signs, symptoms, and lab data into a ranked list of diagnoses that might explain the person's condition. The product has long been a popular electronic teaching tool in medical schools.[38]

Cerner entered this experimental area of medical IT with the *Cerner* Rule System, a solution "carefully crafted with the functionality to evaluate clinical information retrospectively and prospectively as a decision support tool." The system provided support in the areas of clinical quality control, risk management and—like all *Cerner* solutions—cost containment. Twenty conversions took place in the first year after the solution's commercial release, and *Cerner*'s 1990 annual report stated that "already, one institution is saving over $1,000 per day through the 'firing' of a single rule that monitors the accuracy of patient billing."[39]

Cerner's knowledge support solution was renamed *Discern®* in 1991. By that time, the addition of the tool to the company's suite of solutions had already made a big impact on sales. According to the company's 1991 annual report, "this rule-based, expert system was the driving force behind our success in completing comprehensive HNA contracts."[40]

"Rules-based" is a programming technique in which rules represent heuristics, or "rules of thumb," which direct the user to a set of actions to take in a given situation. The two components of a rule are an "if" portion and a "then" portion.[41]

The startling facts about deaths due to medical errors reported in the 1999 paper "To Err Is Human" by the Institute of Medicine had increased public awareness about safety and quality of care, but it did not reverse the harsh statistics. When the report was issued, more than 1 million serious medication errors were occurring every year in U.S. hospitals. Medical errors contributed to 7,000 deaths a year, and the cost of adverse drug events (ADEs) was more than $2 billion a year in hospital costs alone.[42]

Part of the problem may have been due to a 20-year gap between scientific discovery and the routine application of those findings in clinical practice that was described in a 2001 report from the Agency for Healthcare Research and Quality (AHRQ). Hundreds of thousands of research studies are published every year that offer new remedies and approaches that could positively affect care, and the challenge of medical IT is to close that information gap.[43]

The quality problems cited in the AHRQ report included "underuse of services," such as a lack of effective interventions. For example, studies have shown that heart attack patients who receive beta blockers have a 42 percent lower death rate. A study of Medicare recipients revealed, however, that only 21 percent of those eligible received beta blockers.

The life-changing information was not making its way to the ER or critical care physicians. Another quality issue was "overuse of services," such as the extensive use of expensive antibiotics in treating children's ear infections. A study showed that if only half the prescriptions written in a given year had been for a less expensive but equally effective antibiotic, amoxicillin, Colorado's Medicaid program would have saved $400,000.[44]

As the lead federal agency overseeing research designed to improve the quality of care in U.S. hospitals, the AHRQ listed in 2002 several priorities for future research. Included on that list was a call for the industry to "identify effective information technology tools and systems that alert providers in real time to the critical information they need to

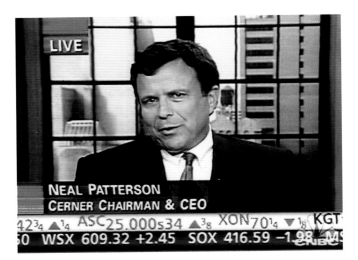

As *Cerner* grew to become a world leader in healthcare IT, CEO Neal Patterson was often called upon to provide an expert voice. In February 1999, he appeared on CNBC to discuss issues within the industry.

provide safer, high-quality care."[45] At *Cerner*, this challenge had been addressed back in 1986 and after years of development resulted in a series of "knowledge-driven" solutions.

Although computers had been used 20 years earlier to assist doctors in accessing published information, *Cerner* developed a system for integrating these knowledge tools seamlessly into solutions that pinpoint the facts, in real time, that a doctor needs to treat a specific person.

According to a company research paper, *Cerner* was "the only HCIT (health care information technology) supplier that delivers this powerful combination—a unified technology platform and industry leading content—to enable knowledge-driven care." These solutions allow the doctor to view a patient's complete medical history and "the best medical evidence before placing an order, effectively closing the healthcare quality loop."[46]

Cerner has developed six solutions in its Knowledge-Driven Care line, including *Discern Expert*®, a rules-based solution based on an extensive database of medical information from Zynx Health, Inc., a subsidiary of Cedars-Sinai Medical Center that *Cerner* acquired in 2002. The Zynx database, considered the industry standard for scientific knowledge and best practices, provided *Cerner* with

an extensive library of clinical rules and evidence-based information surrounding patient safety and regulatory compliance. When embedded in *Discern Expert*®, Zynx ensured that doctors had the information they needed to comply with regulations while making the most informed decisions possible.

"Clinical discoveries or best practices published in a research paper are of little value unless the physician can use the knowledge easily and immediately when caring for patients," said *Cerner* co-founder Paul Gorup when the Zynx acquisition was announced. "*Cerner*'s goal is to close this information loop in healthcare—to increase the amount of new health information that can be incorporated into practice and to condense the amount of time it takes for the knowledge to reach physicians."[47]

Patterson added that Zynx would help *Cerner* take medical IT into a new era:

This is the beginning of a completely new era of information technology in healthcare. Information systems of the future will be defined by how "smart" they are, not only by how well they automate workflow. Zynx has proven its ability to develop and maintain the best available science on how to diagnose and treat a number of human conditions. The only way to get this science into practice is to put only the most relevant information at the physician's fingertips at the point of care. ... Now, we are aligned with the best organization in the world at researching and packaging this science for physician and nurse usage.[48]

Discern Expert® supports decision-making with information in the form of alerts, reminders, order sets, and other compiled knowledge. Caregivers can create, cancel, and add procedures to orders based on evidence-based, quality-controlled guidelines. *Discern Explorer*® and *Executable Knowledge*® are related solutions that offer a variety of database options. Administrators at the University of Illinois Medical Center in Chicago invested in *Discern*® and were pleased by how quickly physicians began using the system.

"With *Discern*®, alerts interact directly with healthcare providers 2,800 times per month," according to a *Cerner* marketing document. "UIMC achieved rapid clinician acceptance of *Executable Knowledge*®. Only six weeks after implementation, alerts triggered change in physician behavior 62 percent of the time."[49]

Cerner divested Zynx Health in 2004 to The Hearst Corporation, one of the largest publishing companies in the world. This move has allowed Zynx content to become more widely deployed within the industry, as more organizations have realized the benefits of evidence-based content in terms of care standardization, reduced care variance and improved care quality. *Zynx Life Sciences*™ was retained in order to further grow *Cerner*'s research and life sciences capabilities.

Cerner addressed the ADE crisis in healthcare with *MediSource*®, released after *Cerner* acquired Multum Information Systems, Inc., in 1998. This solution contains safety checks and reference information that supports order entry, the dispensing of medications from pharmacies, nurse administration, and patient education about their medications. This solution automatically audits the suitability and safety of a drug dose, taking into consideration the person's age, weight, and other factors.

In addition to *MediSource*®, *Cerner* developed a group of rules-based medication solutions that address various areas such as antibiotics, pain management, and cancer therapies. These Medication Utilization and Error Prevention solutions provide clinicians with drug information at the point of care. Also included in this group is the ADE Prevention Alert Foundation package, which notifies a caregiver of a potential ADE before it occurs.

Sun Health Corporation of Sun City, Arizona, developed its own drug safety system around *Cerner*'s ADE Prevention Alert Antibiotic solution. According to Sun Health pharmacist Gary Nechvatal, nurses and clinicians have had a very positive reaction to the automated system.

"The nurses really like the output of the system," he said. "We're able to respond quicker to a lot of the alerts. We get the orders in quicker. And with the patients, we're able to provide the drugs in a much quicker manner, and provide better interaction checking and drug checking."[50]

The solution also made a dramatic impact on the bottom line of the department, with a projected $1 million savings a year on a more efficient method of dosing kidney medication.[51] Based on results from the first months of operation, Sun Health expected a large reduction in ADEs, as well.

"Sun Health predicts that the *Cerner* ADE Prevention Alert Antibiotic Utilization and Error Prevention solution will prevent an average of three ADEs per day," Nechvatal said, "saving the organization between $2.2 and $6 million per year in associated costs."[52]

In 2001, *Cerner* brought its knowledge-driven care solutions to the critical care sector by acquiring APACHE, a company that had created a knowledge database specifically for the ICU. With the database in hand, *Cerner* went on to develop the *Apache III*® solution as a decision support tool that would help

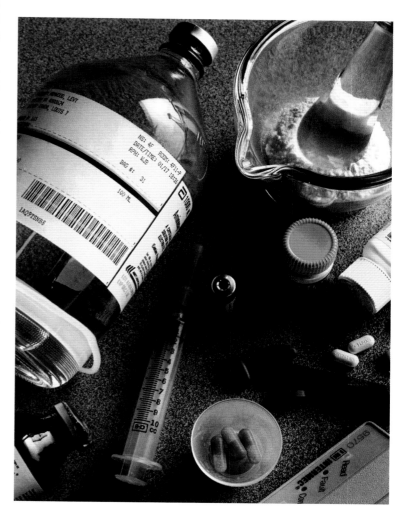

Cerner's pharmacy solution, *PharmNet*®, helps reduce adverse drug events, the medication errors that increase hospital costs by $2 billion a year.

physicians better manage the care of the critically ill. This unique system was based on an enormous pool of data about previous cases that was programmed to predict the most effective therapies for the best possible outcomes.

In its 2001 Annual Report, *Cerner* described the "incredible power" of APACHE's technology:

The APACHE algorithms (logical sequences of steps that can be translated into a computer program) are derived from an empirical database of more than 700,000 actual ICU patient experiences with structured data about their diseases, their treatments, and their outcomes. It has been scientifically proven that these algorithms can predict the outcome of the next patient based on the actual experiences from 700,000 previous cases.[53]

Sarasota Memorial Hospital, an 839-bed trauma center in Florida, was the first hospital in the country to connect the APACHE system directly with a clinical IT system for critical care. Since the conversion to *Apache III*®, Sarasota Memorial has witnessed a steady reduction of ICU and hospital mortality rates. The data provided by the solution has helped clinicians identify specific opportunities for improvement, and clinical nurse specialist Rhonda Anderson, R.N., noted that "this data can be a strong stimulus for change when dealing with physicians."[54]

Even on the most superficial level, *Apache III*® has made Anderson's work easier. "As I make rounds, I also like to see the color screen that reflects acuity and predictions," she said. "A lot of red means higher acuities and much sicker patients. This helps me get an idea of staffing needs."[55]

Cerner also developed a knowledge-driven tool based on data gathered from millions of medical charts nationwide. *Health Facts*® utilizes anonymous and encrypted data to allow users to compare various aspects of their healthcare facility to others in their area or to the industry as a whole, helping to identify areas for quality improvement. The solution also locates and matches people for clinical trials, monitors ADEs, and analyzes trends in care.[56]

Cerner's commitment to this empowering set of solutions has made it the industry leader in knowledge-driven systems. The company continues to inform the industry about facilities that have

made significant improvements in the quality and cost of care after converting to its knowledge-driven solutions, and by late 2004, more than 500 clients had installed these systems.

Cerner co-founder Paul Gorup observed that knowledge-based solutions are gaining more ground among physicians in the new millennium. "I do believe that information-based medicine ... is starting to become more accepted," he said in 2004. "In the last three years, whether it's a critical care doc, chief medical officer or the chief quality officer, they're really pushing it hard. I think the physicians, for the most part, are not fighting it anymore."[57]

Cerner's continuing challenge, according to Gorup, is to make these solutions even more "smart" and simple to use. "What [doctors] are still trying to figure out is, 'How do you make it more proactive versus me either having to pull out the information or me being told I did something wrong?' So we need to tell them what to do before they do it rather than tell them they're ordering the wrong medication after the fact. We need to push out the best options for them so they won't make the mistake."[58]

Specialty Care Solutions Target Specific Areas

In the late 1990s and through 2004, *Cerner* worked on developing groups of solutions tailored to three specialties—women's health, cardiology, and, most recently, oncology. These packages facilitate the conversion of specialty areas to paperless systems, with tailor-made automated solutions that address their particular needs.

Cerner's solutions for women's health include tools for managing everything from fetal monitor data in a maternity ward to the billed charges in a gynecologist's office. *PowerChart for Maternity*®, for example, includes a flowsheet of labor and delivery data, newborn documentation, and newborn growth charts and immunization records. The fetal monitoring solution interfaces with the medical instrument to produce electronic documentation, and the knowledge solutions within the system include decision support rules and reference literature. *OB/Gyn Anesthesia* includes remote monitoring technology, and the *OB Management Dashboard* manages workflow tasks such as patient tracking.

Another set of solutions designed for the obstetrics/gynecology physician's office features a workflow tool that includes prenatal forms and growth charts, and electronic documentation of all office visits. Ob/gyn physicians who use *Cerner*'s solutions can provide concise dating of a woman's gestation with the integrated gestational age calculator, and a woman visiting an office with *Cerner* solutions may find her doctor using a bedside device to instantly record her sonar images into her electronic medical record. Embedded knowledge solutions also give the doctor instant access to scientific and drug information.

Like other *Cerner* solutions, these systems allow the physician to access electronic data from a home office and remain updated about a person's lab results and procedures at all times. Michael Salesin, M.D., a gynecologist at Detroit Medical Center, described the enormous difference this remote capability made in his practice:

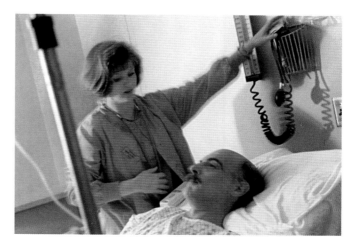

PowerChart Oncology®, a new solution announced in 2004, will help physicians create person-specific cancer treatment plans capable of spanning multiple visits and various treatment locations.

> *It has absolutely changed our whole process. We have immediate access to those reports that, previously, we might not have seen at all. As far as taking care of patients, I'll give you an example. I was concerned about a surgical patient's blood loss at the hospital, and we ordered a blood test. I was able to call in from home and get the results of the blood test very quickly, and then when I called the hospital to speak with the resident about the care of the patient, she was actually surprised that I knew the results before she even had them.*
>
> *Prior to going electronic, we used to have to call the hospital, talk to a clerk, then they called the lab, and we waited for a call back. It might take hours. Sometimes, they just couldn't find the result at all. So it is completely changing our management of patients. The speed with which we can respond to these kinds of results is just amazing.*[59]

With new pressures on cardiology departments to increase patient safety and streamline operations, paper reporting had become increasingly burdensome. In response, *Cerner* designed *CVNet*™ to automate the specific challenges of this area, from a person's initial registration to a broad-based analysis of cardiology procedure outcomes throughout the country. *CVNet*™ allows the cardiologist to

instantly access procedure reports after surgery, and nurses are freed from many tasks because of the solution's ability to automatically create physician referral letters, manage schedules, and generate charges.

This solution is also approved for National Registry Certification, which allows doctors to submit data to a national database and access the registry's information to help the department make decisions about how to improve the quality of care.

In addition to streamlining the operation of cardiology departments, *Cerner*'s electronic medical record gives cardiologists the ability to immediately notify patients of critical information. Cardiologist Anthony Alfieri, M.D., for example, utilized the solution to identify and prescribe alternate medications for people who were impacted by the recall of Baycol, a drug used to reduce the risk of heart disease. Alfieri acknowledged that his practice's former method of paper charting did not begin to measure up to the paperless system.

"Having been on this system for approximately six months, and having been on paper, I can tell you there's no comparison whatsoever," he said. "The fact that we could notify 136 patients in under 24 hours about a dangerous drug is revolutionary."[60]

Another cardiologist emphasized the electronic medical record's value in notifying people about life-or-death issues. Monte Wilson, vice president of Cardiology and Surgical Services at the Sisters of Mercy Health System in St. Louis, Missouri, utilizes the solution during product recall emergencies.

"If there's a recall on a particular implant, we can use the solution to quickly retrieve data on those patients who have received the implants and expeditiously remove the recalled product from our inventory," he said.[61]

Cerner's newest solution, announced in early 2004, focuses on the decision-making and communication needs of cancer care. *PowerChart Oncology*® is being designed specifically for chemotherapy treatment, allowing physicians to create a person-specific treatment plan that can span multiple visits and treatment locations.

The decision-support portion of the solution, *Executable Knowledge for Oncology*, has a database of scientific and clinical information embedded into the physician's online system. *Clinical Trials for Oncology* automates the process of selecting participants for clinical trials by comparing each person's condition to an internal database of the hospital's active trials.

The most cutting-edge aspect of this specialty solution is designed for patients. *IQHealth*™ *Oncology Center* is an electronic format for people with cancer to create a health diary, make updates to a personal health record, schedule visits, and communicate with other patients and clinicians in chat rooms. This solution brings *Cerner* closer to its goal of creating a community-wide, patient-interactive, electronic health network.

Consumer and Community Solutions Put the Person at the Center

One of Patterson's goals for healthcare IT is to put the person at the center of every solution design. "The person—not any enterprise—must be at the center of these architectural models," he wrote in a textbook published in 2004. "Note that this entity is always the person and never the patient." For Patterson, terminology has been a powerful tool in making the paradigm shifts that are necessary to make healthcare more safe and efficient.

"Patient should never be used as a noun, for it is dehumanizing," he wrote. "Patients are sick, vulnerable, and dependent. The person wants to be healthy and independent. Moreover, the word patient fails to acknowledge the lifetime of care the transformed health system will provide."[62]

The "lifetime of care" idea lies at the heart of the company's Consumer and Community Solutions. Patterson envisions systems that go beyond the boundaries of a single hospital or doctor's office. Not only should a person's medical information be accessible throughout his or her lifetime, but throughout the greater system in which the person lives.

"Design the data about the person's health and medical problems to be controlled and managed well beyond the encounter," he wrote.[63]

Cerner's *IQHealth*® solution allows individuals to gain better control of their medical care and expands a person's medical information beyond the traditional boundaries of a clinic, hospital, or physician's office. This solution is connected to a sponsoring Web site, which allows the person to communicate electronically with clinicians to fill out forms, update health information, receive physician referrals, and learn about tailored resources for conditions such as diabetes, asthma, sleep disorders, and congestive heart failure.

The personal health record embedded in the system allows people to update real-time information about their allergies, immunizations, medications, blood pressure, and other aspects of their health. A person with diabetes, for example, can input the results of her home-based blood tests right into her electronic medical record.

As a Web-based communication tool, *IQHealth*® also strengthens the relationship between an individual and his or her healthcare provider. This person-empowered, interactive solution helps fulfill Patterson's vision of a wholly integrated health information community. In the best of all possible worlds, every physician and clinician who has an impact on a person's medical record would have instant access to that record.

"Create a lifelong, secure, personal health record that can be maintained from home, over the Internet," Patterson wrote. "Each interaction with a physician, nurse, pharmacist, laboratory, or technician in the various inpatient, outpatient, home health, public health, and long-term care facilities will contribute something to the personal health record."[64]

Committed to advancing medical care through the personal health record (PHR), *Cerner* launched a groundbreaking program for children with diabetes in the autumn of 2004. The goal of this initiative, to provide every child in the United States with type 1 diabetes a PHR, was backed by a $25 million investment to develop the program over the next 10 years.

Thirteen-thousand children are diagnosed with the disease every year, and the electronic communication provided by *Cerner*'s PHR is designed to cut down on costly office-visit time for those families who can manage the disease well on their own. This will leave more time for doctors to help manage the care of children who have difficulties with their daily regimens and experience more complex medical problems associated with the disease.

According to Lynn B. Nicholas, CEO of the American Diabetes Association, *Cerner*'s program targets the most important goals of her organization. "Core to the mission of the American diabetes Association are two tenets—improve the quality of care, as well as improve the quality of life for people with diabetes," she said. "The initiative planned by *Cerner* has great potential to do both for children with type 1 diabetes and their families."[65]

In addition to Internet-based *IQHealth*®, *Cerner* designed a community solution for the growing home care industry that allows information to be shared electronically from a person's home to the home care or hospice office. In 2003, *Cerner* acquired BeyondNow Technologies, the industry leader in home care information technology, a field that was showing strong growth due to the aging of baby boomers and technological advancements in medicine.

One study estimated that $673 million was spent on IT for home healthcare in 2001 and that those expenditures would grow to $1.4 billion by 2004.[66] With this entrée into the market, *Cerner* was able to enhance a leading product by integrating it with its HNA solutions—and expand its presence in the medical IT industry.

BeyondNow, based in Overland Park, Kansas, was founded in 1994 and had 120 clients when *Cerner* purchased the company. Thirty-two of those companies were already *Cerner* clients or were professionally associated with it. *Cerner* gained two new solutions in this new acquisition: *HomeWorks*®, a complete office management system, and

RoadNotes®, an automated communication system for patient information from the bedside to the office.

Cerner's third solution in this group, *HealthSentry*®, a bioterrorism alert solution, was developed after the attacks of September 11, 2001. "Since the terrorist attacks on September 11, America's medical technology companies have been looking at ways to play a role in our defense against bioterrorism attacks by detecting the symptoms early and treating them more effectively," said Jeff Ezell of the IT trade organization Advanced Medical Technology Associates in Washington, D.C.[67]

Cerner worked with the Kansas City Health Department to develop the solution, which was designed to immediately page health officials if a lab result comes back with a diagnosis of anthrax, plague, or another deadly disease that could be used as a weapon. *HealthSentry*® also monitors infectious diseases in the region, sending the health department daily reports on hundreds of lab tests for people suspected of having an infectious disease.

At a news conference announcing the solution's debut in the spring of 2002, Patterson stated that "our health systems in this country on 9/12 became part of the national defense system," and added that his company aimed to make the Kansas City area "the most well-protected community in the country."[68]

HealthSentry®, developed with the Kansas City Health Department after the 9/11 attacks, was designed to alert healthcare officials whenever a lab result indicates anthrax, plague, or any other disease that can be used as a weapon.

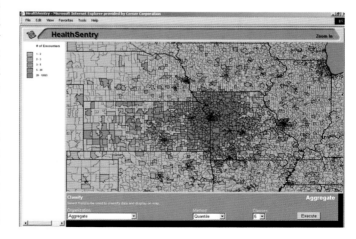

Financial and Operational Solutions
Help Conserve Resources

When *Cerner* entered the medical IT industry in the mid-1980s, a large percentage of the solutions on the market addressed billing and the other financial components of healthcare. The founders did not want to replicate those services and developed a consistent focus on clinical solutions. But as *Cerner* matured, the company's leadership in the industry allowed it to branch into what it referred to as the "surrounding care" portion of healthcare, such as finance, inventory, scheduling, and registration.

A new set of solutions focuses on the revenue cycle of healthcare organizations, something the founders did not think about when they established the company in 1979. But by 2004, according to Steve Oden, vice president of engineering, "it is absolutely the next big footprint for *Cerner*."[69]

Just as the company brought in physicians and other clinicians to build the first *PathNet*® system and all the clinical solutions that followed, the company sought out financial professionals who knew the territory when it began considering a new set of financial solutions.

"I think that it's a completely different mindset for *Cerner* to think about the financial transactions," Oden said. "So we absolutely wanted to bring in people who understood the patient accounting in healthcare, to get CFOs' perspectives."[70]

Cerner's financial solutions were developed in two different groups—*Clinically Driven Revenue Cycle*™ and *Clinically Driven Resource Planning*™. The first group contains solutions that automate billing processes, scheduling, and registration, all of which had been developed as components of other clinical systems.

Cerner had recognized early on that scheduling would be a complex part of its clinical solutions, and Oden recalled putting together a new team to address this aspect of *RadNet*™ when that early solution was being developed. He said:

A big part of RadNet™ *was scheduling patients, taking the calls from the physician's office, and scheduling chest X-rays and MRIs. It soon was apparent that that piece of functionality was a large effort to undertake. We looked at it and said we need to have a separate team focusing on scheduling.*

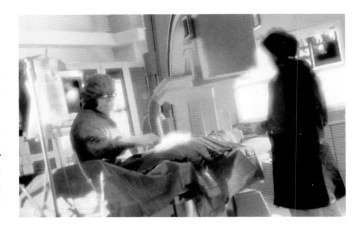

SurgiNet®, released in 1992, helps hospital surgical departments automate tasks related to surgery including the coordination of staff, materials, equipment, locations, and patients. The solution also provides safety alerts, improves inventory management, and streamlines the billing process.

Plus, we had a vision already at that time, Cerner*'s vision of more than just a clinical laboratory. The true HNA vision was starting to take shape. So our vision of scheduling was much more than just "let's get the radiology scheduling done."*[71]

Cerner's five *CapStone*® solutions are the most advanced incarnation of the company's long-term commitment to the scheduling aspect of healthcare. *CapStone*® addresses scheduling and registration; the *ProFile*® *Health Information Management System* is a coding and electronic medical record solution; *Medical Transcription Management* automates transcription services; and the *ProFit*™ *Enterprise Billing and Accounts Receivable System* addresses patient accounting.

The *Clinically Driven Resource Planning*™ set of financial solutions provides automated systems for staff scheduling, for matching patients with appropriate clinicians in a healthcare facility, and for analyzing the organization's use of staff and materials. *Cerner* also developed two enterprise-wide solutions in this group that address the big-picture needs of administrators.

PowerInsight® transforms the combined clinical, operational, and financial data of an organization into a data warehouse that can be used to manage the overall operation of the facility. The information empowers managers to reduce costs, improve care, and increase patient safety. Competitors' products use this approach to analyze one business issue at a time, while *Cerner's* solution analyzes every level of the organization. This structure makes *Cerner's* solution "the most robust data warehouse and healthcare intelligence solution in the industry."[72]

"*PowerInsight®* [helps clinicians] manage their business by being able to drill down and see what's happening in their organization, both clinically and tying it to financial data," said Shellee Spring, vice president of grid services. "Right now, there's no one in the market that can do all that to be able to give you such relevant data. You can also take that to the discrete level … to do costing, which no one can do either, because they don't have the discrete data that we have."[73]

The second enterprise-wide solution, *Cerner's ProVision® Document Image Management System*, was introduced to the market at the 2001 meeting of the Radiological Society of North America. This technology embeds every image pertaining to a person's care into the electronic medical record. "*ProVision®* is unique in the industry because it already delivers comprehensive integration between the image archives and the clinical information system," a *Cerner* press release stated.[74]

Cerner President Trace Devanny explained that "an electronic medical record isn't complete unless it can contain all types of images. Clinicians need to have the complete picture to provide proper and timely care. *Cerner ProVision®* integrates these images into the electronic medical record permanently. This includes all clinical images, whether they come from radiology, cardiology, oncology, or other areas of the hospital."[75]

Forging into the financial realm of healthcare IT brought the three *Cerner* founders full circle to their Andersen Consulting days, when they used software to solve business problems for a wide variety of firms, from tax preparation experts to trucking companies. Once they focused on medical IT in their own firm, however, the company became the leading supplier of healthcare IT in the nation and the world. Every decision about development has remained consistent to that vision and allowed the company to grow.

"Not only did the vision set a good linear target for us," said Oden, "we've actually been able to grow our vision almost horizontally so that it continues to encompass more and more of what's important to healthcare. That's got to be one of the keys to the success of that vision." Oden continued:

> It was a very evolutionary-tolerant vision. It allowed us to drive our company early on, and then it allowed us to branch and continue to build upon it to where we created the company we have today. So it's scale, and it's scope, and it's the fact that vision could grow with healthcare and stay relevant and drive a business that continued to succeed and grow along with it.[76]

Cerner Vice President and Chief Architect Chris Murrish, who joined the company in 1986, recognized that *Cerner's* expansion into many aspects of healthcare was inevitable, even though the original focus was on the lab. There was resistance to Patterson's vision at times, as Murrish explained, but the company's wide base of solutions was in line with everything the company had envisioned since Murrish's first year. He said:

> We could have taken the safe route and stayed in our niche area in the lab, but I don't think we'd have survived. We wouldn't be here today. So Neal, being the visionary that he was, knew that we had to go out. Some of us resisted. We were happy in the lab area. We thought moving into radiology and pharmacy was too much to handle with the staff that we had. We weren't that big of a company. Certainly it turns out we had to do that.[77]

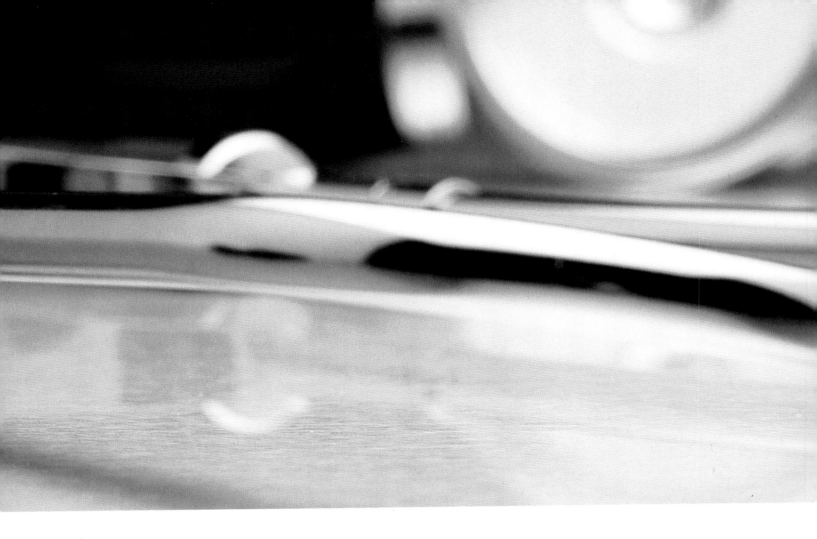

MILESTONES

1995
Cerner Health Conference attracts record 750 attendees. First Hand Foundation is established.

1996
Cerner 2000 initiative is launched. Partnership with Siemens expands global presence.

1999
Cerner celebrates 20th anniversary, makes *Fortune* list of "Best 100 Companies to Work For."

2000
Company becomes charter member of The Leapfrog Group to help reduce medical mistakes.

INTELLECTUAL PROPERTY DEVELOPMENT

1993
Company begins making plans for new architecture.

1995
Apache Medical Systems are incorporated into *Cerner* solutions. *Cerner* Vision Center II opens.

1996
Company launches *Cerner* Virtual University.

1999
HNA Millennium Phase I is completed.

GROWTH

1994
1,000 associates. *Cerner* buys Rockcreek Office Park.

1995
Secondary stock offering raises $100 million.

1997
2,000 associates.

1999
Company partners with Synetic (now called WebMD), Ernst & Young, and Arthur Andersen.

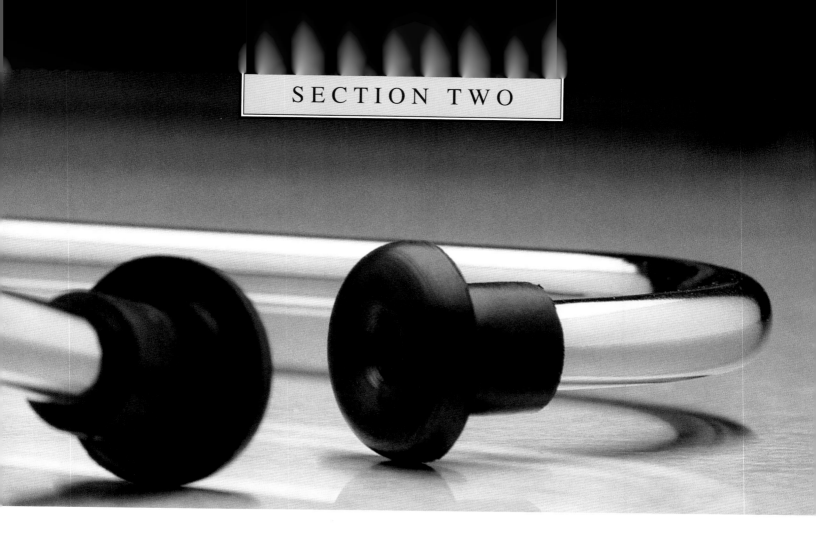

SECTION TWO

001
eptember 11 terrorist attacks
ke place, prompting design of
oterrorism solution.

2003
Company reorganizes into five
Cerner in *Cerner* (CinC) regions.

2004
Cerner celebrates 25th anniversary.

2005
Cerner ranks third amongst software
companies in the *Wall Street Journal*'s
Top 50 Returns over a five-year period.

999
2K watch includes 24-hour service
osts set up two days prior and one
y after the new year.

2000
IQHealth is launched. Winona Health
Online connects an entire Minnesota
town. Pocket *PowerChart®* debuts.

2003
2,649 Millennium solutions online
at 567 facilities.

2004
Lighthouse solutions in development
harvest healthcare methodologies and
deliver them to clients.

02
000 associates.

2003
Cerner awarded U.K. National Health
Service's Choose and Book contract.

2004
Cerner launches the Bedrock initiative,
drastically reducing system implementation time and overall costs.

2005
Cerner awarded NHS contract in England.
Company launches statewide Tennessee
health record.

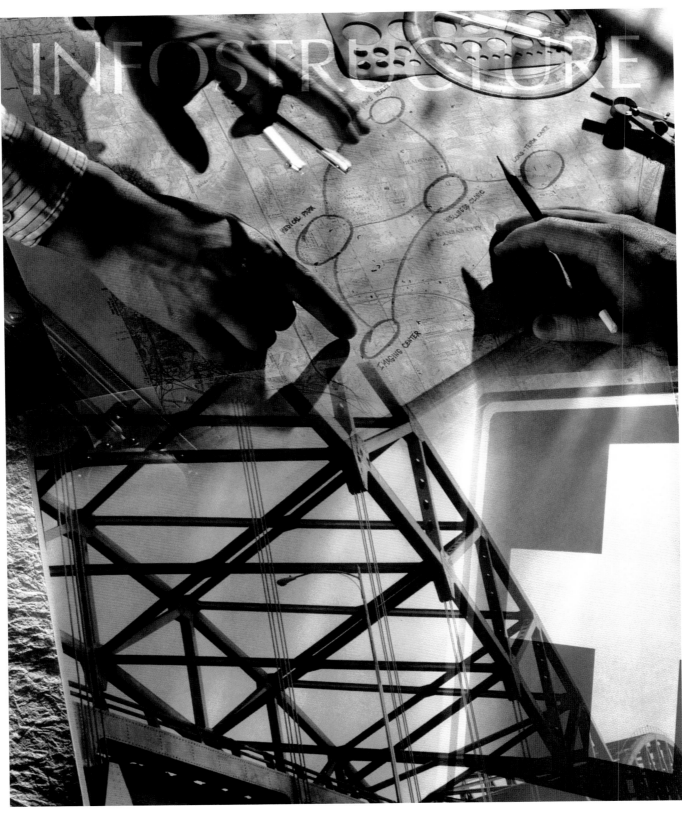

As the new millennium approached, *Cerner* committed itself to a courageous, visionary—and expensive—plan to reinvent the company's architecture, creating a person-centered system.

CHAPTER SIX

A NEW MILLENNIUM

By then we were absolutely convinced that the logical information center for the practice of medicine was the person, from the moment of conception to the moment of death, in illness and in health, and in healthcare contexts from the operating room to the living room. Anything else ... was a compromise. In version 500, we were going to make the major shift that would allow us to build the relational data model our vision demanded.

—Neal Patterson, *Cerner* co-founder and CEO[1]

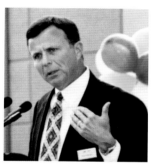

THE TURBULENT END OF THE 20th century has brought new challenges for *Cerner*, from the threat of a Y2K disaster to the stark new realities of terrorism in the post-9/11 world. *Cerner* has approached these challenges with its now-legendary commitment to innovation. At the heart of this commitment was a courageous plan, mapped out in the early 1990s, to completely reinvent the company's architecture from the "classic" Health Network Architecture (HNA) to HNA Millennium, a design that has paved the way for healthcare IT in the 21st century.

Betting the Company

From 1990 to 1994, *Cerner* enjoyed a period of solid growth with a broad line of solutions built on its HNA system—called V300 at the time—as well as its successful *PowerChart®* solution, described by Patterson as "healthcare's first real commercially available electronic medical record."[2] During that time, lead architects David McCallie and Margaret Kolm of *Cerner*'s Boston headquarters, also known as *Cerner* East, developed the company's Open Clinical Foundation (OCF) group of solutions, known as V400.

Even though the V400 version of the architecture was a significant leap forward, Patterson knew that more needed to be done to keep up with the direction that IT was headed. A fifth version of HNA was inevitable, and it would require much more than an upgrade of V400. The future, according to Patterson, demanded a completely new system that would put *Cerner*'s engineers back at square one.

Patterson began laying the groundwork for this new architecture in December 1993 after all the attendees had left the *Cerner* Health Conference. Patterson sat down at the Italian Gardens restaurant in Kansas City with Gay Johannes to discuss *Cerner*'s vision and the technical possibilities of a new architecture. Johannes, who was responsible for *PathNet®* at the time, had started at the company as a programmer in 1983. That conversation helped Patterson formulate his ideas about a commitment to the future of healthcare IT that would incur substantial costs.

"The thought of initiating ... a project and an architecture that would over time replace the V300 and V400 solution sets was daunting to almost all of us," Patterson said. "But we knew that it was what we had to do because our future was at stake."[3]

CEO Neal Patterson realized early on that the only way for *Cerner* to keep up with the direction healthcare IT was heading was to build a new architecture from scratch.

After exploring the idea with Johannes, Patterson followed up with software engineer Bryan Ince, another associate who had been developing solutions since 1983. In January 1994, Patterson and Ince sat at a table at The Bristol—the now-legendary hangout where the founders had brainstormed to create *PathNet*®—and sketched the original design for a new architecture, code-named Tablerock.[4]

Ince accepted Patterson's challenge and put together a small team consisting of associates Laurie Bohlman, David Edwards, Tom Hanf, Matt Hodes, Doug McNair, Chris Murrish, Mike Schmitt, and Owen Straub. Each member of the team, led by Ince and Jeff Townsend, was an experienced engineering architect who had already worked on major solutions for *Cerner*. The project was kept under wraps at first; the team itself would need time to get comfortable with the radical idea of reinventing and rewriting the *Cerner* architecture and all of its solutions. Ince set up his group in a small, isolated room on the sixth floor of the 2900 building.

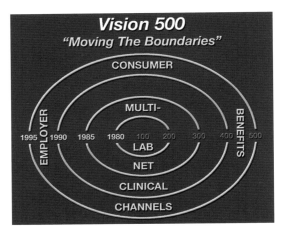

"We tried to keep it small," said Ince. "We tried to keep it somewhat secret.… We put up a … hidden, mysterious room with no windows in it. People didn't necessarily know what was going on in there."[5]

In brainstorming sessions in the "hidden" room and at The Depot Saloon in Avondale, just north of *Cerner* headquarters, Patterson and the Tablerock team sketched out designs for the new system on tablets and paper napkins. The project was soon renamed V500, then HNA Millennium, as the group developed the new architecture. In this "war room" environment, which had spread to the sixth and seventh floors of the 2900 building, more than 200 software developers and people with related roles worked for just over two years to streamline communication and transfer technical and functional knowledge.

"The outcome," said Patterson, "was a healthcare information technology architecture unmatched for its capabilities and for its potential to drive the transformation of healthcare around the world."[6]

This demand for a new architecture was based on two healthcare issues: the need for a medical IT solution that addressed both business and clinical areas; and the benefits of a person-centered system that operated throughout the entire continuum of care, from the home to the hospital and every clinical site in between.[7] According to Patterson, an architecture that delivered these capabilities was the only kind that could function in the future.

In the early years of the company, Patterson realized that technology would one day be able to support the person-centered approach he envisioned. David McCallie, *Cerner*'s vice president of medical informatics and chief scientist, explained that the smaller databases during the early days of healthcare IT stored a person's information for only about 45 days, after which it would be erased to make room for new data.

"When you talk about a patient-centered system, it's really only concerned about the data being available while [the person is] a patient," McCallie said. "But a person-centered system says they're going to come back some day, so let's keep this data online and make it a permanent record."[8]

McCallie further explained how Patterson's prediction of more storage capacity came to fruition as *Cerner* grew:

Neal likes to say, "Being a patient is a status." You're a person now, but you might be a patient again next year. So the data repository that OCF, the Open Clinical Foundation, became was designed to hold a permanent, lifetime record of information about this person regardless of whether they happen

Cerner's new architecture, once called V500, was envisioned as a flexible system that would allow information to be shared at every level of care, from the lab to the consumer.

to be a patient right now or not. The traditional design assumed 45 days, and the data was going to get purged, whereas OCF said, we're going to keep it forever. You're going to have to buy more disks to put in your computer, but it will just grow forever, and we won't ever purge it.

So that was a fundamental shift that needed new technology, new thinking, new hardware capabilities. When I joined Cerner in 1991, a gigabyte of disk storage was $1,000. Today, … a gigabyte is less than a dollar. So there has been a thousand-fold improvement in storage capacity over the course of the 13 years I've been at Cerner, and without that, you couldn't do what we wanted to do, but we knew that would happen. We knew that the technology would just continue to evolve.[9]

The transformation from Classic to Millennium would involve not only a new type of programming and software technology, but a heavy investment in research and development.

One of the members of the Tablerock team, Owen Straub, recalled the gravity of the challenge that Patterson put before him and the rest of the group during its first meetings. "Neal reflected and said, 'I think we're going to have to start over.'" Straub said. "Basically, the phrase he used with us was, 'We're going to bet the company.'" Straub continued:

You realize that all of our code was over in a different technology. At the time it was COBOL, RNS file systems, and we needed to be someplace else. Neal … realized that, over time, we'll be dead on the technology that we have. So he used the words "bet the company" with us in that meeting…. Everybody is sitting around the table. We're going, "Thanks, Neal, you just put a huge challenge on us."[10]

During the mid-1990s, *Cerner* made an enormous financial investment in HNA Millennium, with cash spending for research and development reaching $43 million by 1996. Because Millennium had not been brought to the marketplace, the focus on the new architecture took a toll on the company's bottom line.

As the 1997 annual report explained, "During 1996, our marketing efforts were adversely impacted because we had committed the bulk of our talent to HNA Millennium, and it was not yet demonstra-

ble in a production setting or generating revenue."[11] In other words, Patterson and his engineering team truly *had* bet the company. The immediate consequences for shareholders were severe.

Patterson, right, with co-founder Cliff Illig in 1993, told members of the Tablerock team in the early 1990s that they were going to "bet the company" on developing a brand-new architecture, HNA Millennium.

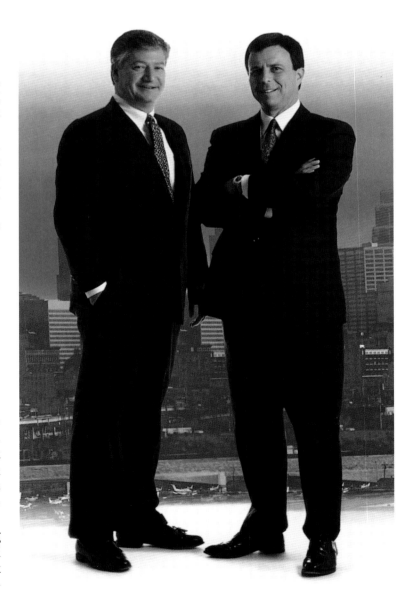

BALANCED BUDGET ACT ROCKS HEALTHCARE

IN 1997, THE U.S. CONGRESS PASSED A law that dramatically changed Medicare, the government's health insurance program for people age 65 and older and disabled individuals. The change came because lawmakers were forced to reduce the cost of this giant federal program, the cost of which had doubled between 1975 and 1995. In 1995 Medicare accounted for 11.3 percent of the entire federal budget.[1]

The Balanced Budget Act (BBA) was designed to create savings of $112 billion to $170 billion over five years by decreasing payments made to physicians, hospitals, and other healthcare providers. The cuts to hospitals included payments for care, as well as for capital expenses.

The industry's initial attempts to deal with reduced Medicare payments resulted in widespread chaos and mass layoffs. In 1999, Patterson reflected on the turmoil that the BBA had brought to the healthcare industry during that decade:

> *Healthcare has fundamentally changed drastically during the '90s, and those changes have accumulated and really are compounding themselves right now. The most recent set of events with the Balanced Budget Act has done nothing but put huge pressures on the industry by taking out a whole bunch of capital and operating margins that would have been there had we not enacted that legislation. So we have an industry that is really now under huge stress. They're scared. I'm in a couple industry groups where almost anyplace you look, about a third to half of the people have been basically let go. So there's chaos out there in the market we sell into.[2]*

In the longer term, however, the Balanced Budget Act was a wake-up call that would ultimately help the industry to understand the benefits of medical IT. The vast reduction in payments for Medicare-related healthcare forced hospitals and other facilities to streamline their operations and find cost savings wherever they could. Many came to realize that although the capital investment in *Cerner*'s enterprise-wide solutions was large, the cost-saving effects of these solutions would deliver results in both the short and long term.

Note this is a hand enrollment pursuant to Public Law 105–32.

H. R. 2015

One Hundred Fifth Congress
of the
United States of America

AT THE FIRST SESSION

*Begun and held at the City of Washington on Tuesday,
the seventh day of January, one thousand nine hundred and ninety-seven*

An Act

To provide for reconciliation pursuant to subsections (b)(1) and (c) of section 105 of the concurrent resolution on the budget for fiscal year 1998.

Be it enacted by the Senate and House of Representatives of the United States of America in Congress assembled,

SECTION 1. SHORT TITLE.

This Act may be cited as the "Balanced Budget Act of 1997".

SEC. 2. TABLE OF TITLES.

This Act is organized into titles as follows:

Title I—Food Stamp Provisions
Title II—Housing and Related Provisions
Title III—Communications and Spectrum Allocation Provisions
Title IV—Medicare, Medicaid, and Children's Health Provisions
Title V—Welfare and Related Provisions
Title VI—Education and Related Provisions
Title VII—Civil Service Retirement and Related Provisions
Title VIII—Veterans and Related Provisions
Title IX—Asset Sales, User Fees, and Miscellaneous Provisions
Title X—Budget Enforcement and Process Provisions
Title XI—District of Columbia Revitalization

TITLE I—FOOD STAMP PROVISIONS

SEC. 1001. EXEMPTION.

Section 6(o) of the Food Stamp Act of 1977 (7 U.S.C. 2015(o)) is amended—
    (1) in paragraph (2)(D), by striking "or (5)" and inserting "(5), or (6)";
    (2) by redesignating paragraph (6) as paragraph (7); and
    (3) by inserting after paragraph (5) the following:
    "(6) 15-PERCENT EXEMPTION.—
      "(A) DEFINITIONS.—In this paragraph:
        "(i) CASELOAD.—The term 'caseload' means the average monthly number of individuals receiving food stamps during the 12-month period ending the preceding June 30.
        "(ii) COVERED INDIVIDUAL.—The term 'covered individual' means a food stamp recipient, or an individual denied eligibility for food stamp benefits solely due to paragraph (2), who—
          "(I) is not eligible for an exception under paragraph (3);

For the first time in eight years, *Cerner* experienced a decrease in earnings in 1996. Net earnings dropped from $22.5 million in 1995 to $8.25 million, and earnings per share plummeted from $.72 to $.25. The company explained the drop in earnings, due to heavy investment in research and development, in its annual report:

> *This allowed competitors to make uncharacteristic inroads into the market for integrated Health Information Systems, a market that* Cerner *led in the first half of the 1990s. While our sales performance was less than planned, we made a deliberate decision to keep building our organization by restructuring and increasing the size of our sales organization, increasing product development capabilities, and increasing infrastructure spending to nearly $120 million, compared with $97 million in the previous year.*[12]

Patterson, who was willing to risk slow sales in the short term to advance *Cerner*'s greater vision, had complete faith in Millennium. He was confident that the future of healthcare IT demanded this revolutionary change. In 1993, he wrote:

> *By then we were absolutely convinced that the logical information center for the practice of medicine was the person, from the moment of conception to the moment of death, in illness and in health, and in healthcare contexts from the operating room to the living room. Anything else, even the "patient," was a compromise. In version 500, we were going to make the major shift that would allow us to build the relational data model our vision demanded.*[13]

Brian Streich, director of intellectual property, recalled some of the questions that surrounded the development of the person-centered approach: "How do we manage the healthcare of that person, versus provide tools and systems for the hospital? From cradle to grave, is my health being managed? Am I tracking all the things I need to track, making healthier people, which ends up costing less for either the consumer or the company that's paying the bills, from an insurance company or the state or the hospitals themselves? We were working that out."[14]

Even though *Cerner*'s stock price stumbled throughout 1996, the company was headed for an even greater leadership position in the industry with its new architecture. Described by one former *Cerner* board member as a "marathon strategy" rather than a sprint, the transition to HNA Millennium would give *Cerner* a solid position in the future of healthcare.

In December 1996, *Kansas City Star* business reporter Julius Karash wrote, "Despite the fact that *Cerner* stock has languished over the last 12 months, analysts say new software and a beefed-up sales force are positioning *Cerner* for long-term growth in the exploding healthcare information industry."[15]

While *Cerner* invested in this long-term growth, other IT companies were buying up businesses to increase their value in the short term. Tablerock team director Jeff Townsend, current chief of staff and executive vice president, recalled one company that thrived during this period. "While we were trying to build this thing from the ground up, McKesson (HBOC at the time) was out buying companies and creating roll-ups, and their stock was doing great, and they were growing like gangbusters, but they're not at the heart of solving the problems," he said.[16]

Cerner, on the other hand, was committed to meeting the challenges the industry demanded. "The core, what we were selling our clients at the time and what we believed in, was this integration," Townsend said. "The lab wants to know what the nurse knows. The nurse wants to know what's going on in the pharmacy. That's where we were unique. We were the only ones in the industry that tried to build the breadth. Everybody else was doing acquisitions."[17]

Cerner's innovative new architecture set it apart from the competition and was recognized by the industry as a groundbreaking development. Dick Brown, co-chairman of the board for the Stowers Institute for Medical Research, recognized *Cerner*'s leadership in the field through its "commitment to build an integrated architecture that ultimately allows the lab, the pharmacy, the radiology departments to all have a common view of what's happening with the medical record, as opposed to the stand-alone departmental systems that preceded an integrated architecture thought."[18]

Unlike the competition, *Cerner*'s architecture was truly integrated. Brown said, "To build most of this from the ground up so that it does integrate— as opposed to going out and acquiring a cats-and-dogs kind of array of companies and sticking them together and claiming to have an integrated health-care systems architecture—represents the implementation of the vision from a very high level of a very complicated, transaction-heavy business enterprise, the hospital."[19]

Tim Zoph, CIO of Northwestern Memorial Hospital in Chicago, described how Cerner's commitment to innovation impressed his facility.

"To Cerner's credit, in '95, they took the long view and said, architectures matter. Integrated information systems matter. The idea that you're going to put the patient or the person at the center matters. So they actually, very early on ... bet the company on an integrated architecture. We liked that sort of strong vision, very purposeful thinking around how the patient experience needs to be automated."[20]

HNA Millennium Innovations

With HNA Millennium, Cerner set the stage for a person-centric healthcare IT system. Patterson knew that the mainframe structure, upon which HNA Classic and competitors' IT systems were based, was not flexible enough to connect all the elements of the healthcare community to each other.

Millennium introduced a new element into the client/server model of computing, upgrading it from a two-tier to a three-tier system, also known in the industry as an "n-tier" system. The client/server model processes data between clients and servers on a network, and assigns a function to the machine best suited to perform the task. The client segment of the model resides on the user's computer, and the server segment is the remote system to which the client's request is sent.[21]

Millennium was designed as an alternative to the traditional approach of intertwining various stand-alone applications, which can be compared to building a house in which rooms are designed by different architects and wired separately with various types of security systems. In a two-tiered client/server system, the user interface (the user's method of interacting with the system) is stored in the client's computer, the data is stored in the server, and the application logic (the system's circuit design and principles) can be stored in either location.

Cerner's three-tiered architecture stores the user interface in the client's computer, the data in a database server, and the majority of the business application logic in one or more additional servers. Millennium also incorporates advanced "messaging middleware," which enables applications to communicate with each other in real time.[22] This new three-tiered system enhances the speed, reliability, and flexibility of the client/server model.

The benefits of this architecture included an easy-to-use desktop interface; increased scalability, speed, and security; and support for mobile, hand-held devices. Designed to run on personal computers (PCs) using Windows 95 or Windows NT Workstation operating systems, Millennium took Cerner solutions to the user-friendly graphical desktop. Users could easily customize and personalize their desktop interface with the now-standard graphical-user interface, which replaced the green-screen, DOS (Disk Operating System) computer system that had been in use since the 1950s.

The increased scalability of the system allows organizations to scale their computer systems to match their business strategies and rate of growth. Hospitals, clinics and physicians' offices of all sizes can rescale horizontally (adding or removing computers on the network) and vertically (upgrading processing performance) without experiencing long periods of downtime or incurring the expense of reengineering the entire system. This feature allows facilities to invest in a cutting-edge system at their own pace.

Millennium improves the speed of computing by processing data across multiple computers simultaneously. With Cerner's long-term vision of entire connected communities, security is also a core focus of the new architecture's design. The company created the most secure automation process in the industry by integrating a variety of confidentiality levels within the data; restricting certain users on a "need-to-know" basis; and incorporating authentication, encryption, and other security mechanisms.[23]

The first level of security involves authentication, which identifies valid users. The second area is access control, a set of permissions that allows the user to access the system.

"The third area that often gets overlooked is auditing or accountability, which can detect what things you do in the system," said John Travis, director of solution management for revenue cycle management. "I can track the ways that you access

HNA MILLENNIUM
HEALTH NETWORK ARCHITECTURE

patient records. I know what records you touch and what operations you did on them."[24]

The system can create a report to alert management about suspicious activity, such as someone downloading files of information on all patients who take a particular drug, for example.[25]

In addition, the architecture was designed to address the new wave of mobile computing and is compatible with all types of point-of-care equipment, such as handheld radio-frequency (RF) devices. With Millennium, information from mobile handheld devices, barcode scanners, optical readers, and speech recognition systems is channeled directly to the network, which then sends the data to the server.

Millennium solutions were also designed to provide operational benefits for the organization,

Above: The benefits of Millennium include increased scalability, speed, and security.

Below: Millennium advanced the client/server model of information technology to a three-tiered system.

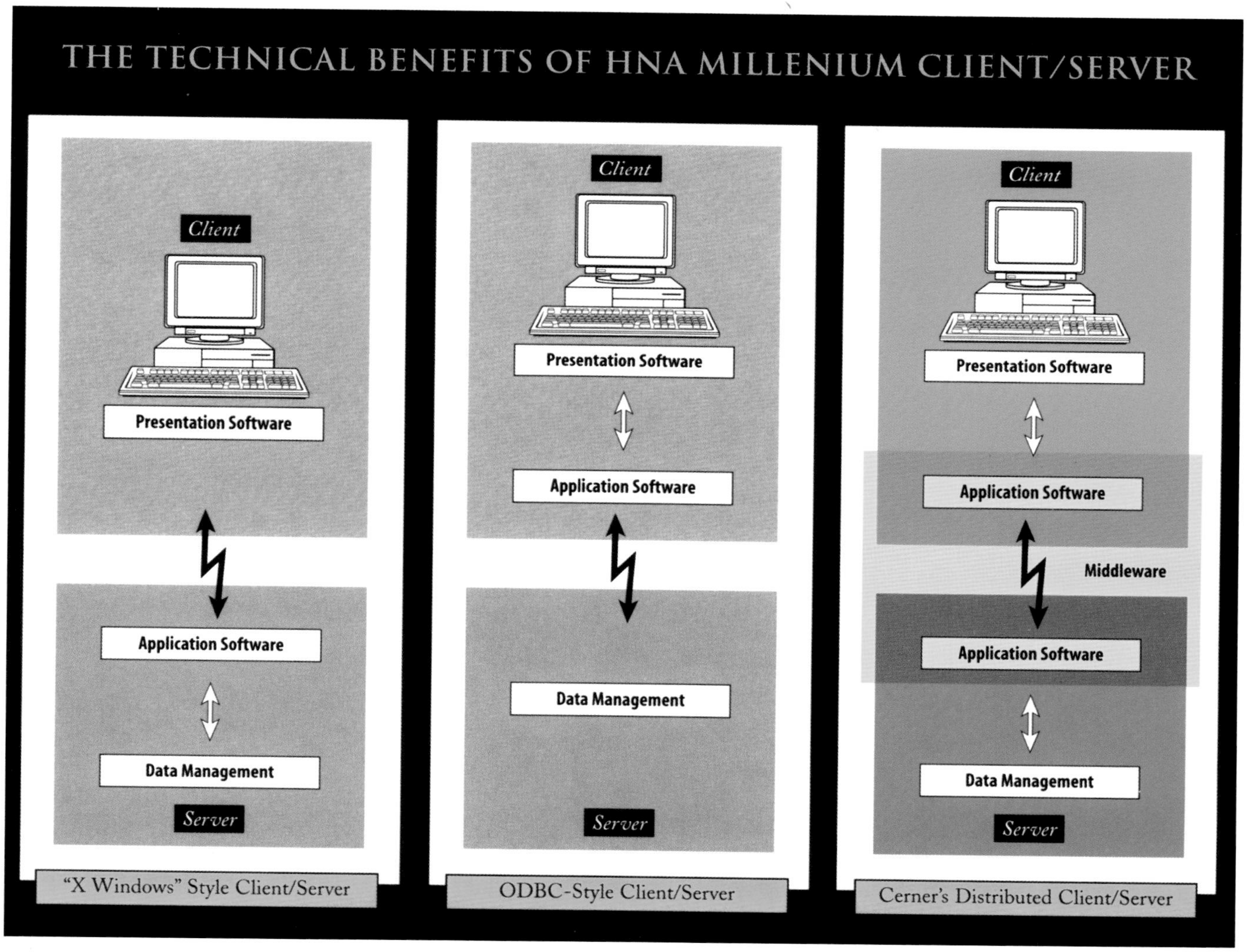

THE TECHNICAL BENEFITS OF HNA MILLENIUM CLIENT/SERVER

Client

Presentation Software

Application Software

Data Management

Server

"X Windows" Style Client/Server

Client

Presentation Software

Application Software

Data Management

Server

ODBC-Style Client/Server

Client

Presentation Software

Application Software

Middleware

Application Software

Data Management

Server

Cerner's Distributed Client/Server

such as measuring performance and identifying best practices. The architecture allows the facility to monitor clinical outcomes, which paves the way for making adjustments in procedures to make the clinic or hospital as efficient as possible. Another cost-effective benefit of the architecture is its ability to run on modern, affordable, faster, and more powerful PCs, which are much less expensive than the mainframes used with older IT systems.

With plans to add a Web-based server element to Millennium, *Cerner* is working to offer its clients an even more versatile and efficient sys-

tem. Designed around the top usability issues that clients have voiced to the company, Millennium's Web-based extension is being designed to increase the ease of navigation, speed, and connectivity of *Cerner* solutions.

Navigation is enhanced by eliminating many of the mouse clicks that take a user to various locations within the system, creating what *Cerner* calls the "ideal experience." Speed, or performance, is improved by transporting the user's requests and replies to and from the database more quickly. The third usability issue, connectivity, pertains to the power of a Web-based Millennium system to connect users through mobile devices. A physician, for example, can place an order for medication from his cell phone if a patient requests it when he is away from the office or hospital. Via Millennium's secure Web connection, the physician can make the call to the pharmacy while the patient is still on the phone.

The Web-based element of Millennium is designed to work as an add-on to existing Millennium

---

Inset: Millennium, *Cerner*'s new architecture, brings wireless technology to the bedside with solutions that can operate on various mobile devices.

Below: The first Millennium conversion took place in 1997 at Integris Baptist Medical Center in Oklahoma City. *(Photo courtesy of Integris Baptist Medical Center.)*

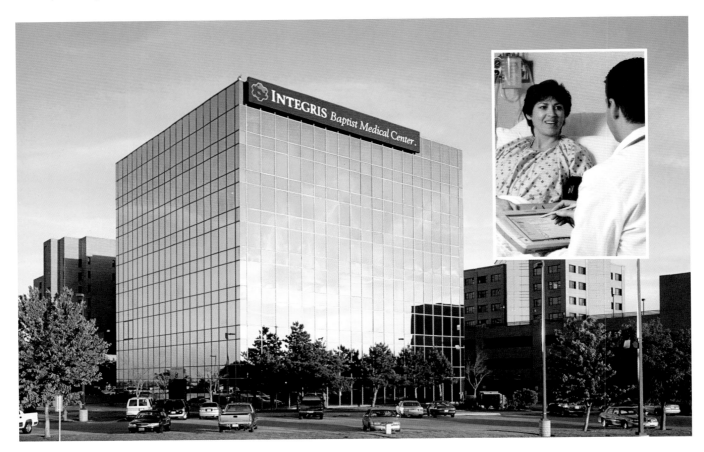

systems and does not require modifications to any *Cerner* solutions. Clients who have invested heavily in converting from *Cerner* Classic to Millennium solutions are assured that their investment is protected. The architecture itself has not changed with the introduction of a Web-based element; rather, it provides another "pipe" through which to access the architecture's powerful back end. The flexible nature of the technology's front end allows clients to access Millennium's back end through a PC or the World Wide Web, or both.

Whichever type of Millennium connection the client uses, the new architecture provides greater efficiency, with the ability to uncover a single invoice or electrocardiogram in seconds; mouse-click inputs and commands that eliminate the need to type; and quick Internet access.[26]

The new client/server model of Millennium has made an enormous impact on the industry. "A physician executive described it to me by saying that the old mainframe systems are like robots," said Jake Sorg, president of *Cerner* Mid-America. "You turn them on. You program them to do something, and they just do the same thing over and over again, versus the relational database in Millennium in the three-tiered client/server world. It's like a patient. It's going to change and react to different stimuli, and you have to be vigilant to that."[27]

Following the most intense development period for Millennium in 1995 and 1996, the new architecture was converted at two alpha sites in 1997. This conversion phase was very costly. By the time the entire set of Millennium solutions was online in various facilities at the beginning of the new century, the company had invested a fortune in research and development.

"I think it was a lot harder than we ever would have guessed," said *Cerner* President Trace Devanny. "It took us longer, [cost] more money. We made our competitors very happy there for a while. Made Wall Street very curious about what we were doing."[28]

Devanny added that the scale of *Cerner*'s challenge was enormous, and the result would have a major impact on the healthcare industry. "It was one of the largest, most complex IT projects in history," he said. "It's very complex to build, very complex to troubleshoot, and very complex to successfully deploy because the problems that our clients are wrestling with are very complex problems."[29]

Implementing HNA Millennium

When the Millennium software engineering team outgrew its small space in the 2900 building at *Cerner* headquarters, the group's directors decided to set up a work space that would closely resemble an actual client site. Through past experience, *Cerner* executives knew that the client site is where all the real work gets done. "Our history had always told us whenever we tried to do something really hard, we succeeded when we got close to the client," Townsend said.[30]

The alpha site for Millennium was in Oklahoma City, but flying hundreds of associates back and forth every week would be costly in both dollars and time. The solution came when some tenants left the 2900 building, and two entire floors opened up. "Instead of building those out with offices and cubes, we just rolled out carpet and put up folding tables," Townsend said. "Every person got a table and a half. So we had two floors that had probably [hundreds of] people each."[31]

From this setting, day-to-day development, as well as testing and documentation, in support of Millennium conversions was conducted.

Each floor, covered with hundreds of programmers and clinicians, represented the working space at a hospital, where a team of associates would usually be relegated to a basement or other large unused area to work on cast-off tables and broken chairs. Without room dividers or cubes, each associate could easily find someone in the room to help answer questions and give advice. Townsend used the model of a grocery store, hanging signs from the ceiling that identified the teams. Anyone walking onto the floor could easily find the "Lab," "Nursing," "Physicians," and other areas of the project.

"You'd get off the elevator at that floor and see a sea of humanity cranking on code and people talking back and forth to each other, yelling across the floor," Townsend said.[32]

A unique feature of each floor was a system that alerted engineers when a server crash occurred and the system went down temporarily. Rather than using pagers, which the company believed caused too many unwanted interruptions, this system—modeled after the blue light used at K-Mart stores to alert shoppers of special deals—utilized a blinking blue light set up in clear view of the entire room.

25 YEARS OF INNOVATION

BY 2004, THE YEAR OF *CERNER*'S 25TH anniversary, the company had grown to become the undisputed leader of health-care information technology with 3,098 *Cerner* Millennium solutions live at 642 facilities.[1]

What began as a discussion on the future of healthcare at a picnic table in Loose Park, Kansas City, had evolved into an almost $1 bil-lion company employing more than 5,000 asso-ciates worldwide.[2]

In these brainstorming sessions, Neal Patter-son, Cliff Illig, and Paul Gorup would consider the advice given to them by Ewing Kauffman, the legendary pharmaceutical billionaire and former owner of the Kansas City Royals:

Treat those who work for the company with respect; call them associates rather than employ-ees; hold regular town hall meetings; offer stock options; and fight to knock out bureaucracy, complacency, and hierarchy.[3]

Upon *Cerner*'s 25th anniversary, associates celebrated by reflecting back on what had contributed to *Cerner*'s overwhelming success. Some recognized the founding fathers' spirit of risk, which was vital in creating an innovative environment that encouraged associates to constantly strive for improvement.

Others singled out the company's commit-ment to research and development. Between 1995 and 2004, *Cerner*'s investment in research and development totaled more than $1 billion or 21 percent of revenue, more than any other in the industry.[4]

Yet it may have been the relevancy of *Cerner*'s vision for creating a healthcare system organized around the individual, not the encounter, which has sustained its status at the top.

As the country's largest independent health-care technology company, *Cerner* has undoubtedly earned a voice in future discussions over health-care at a national level.

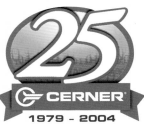

Below left: Marking *Cerner*'s 25th anniversary on September 4, 2004, from left to right, Neal Patterson, Paul Gorup, and Cliff Illig remi-nisce with associates. Below right: A group of longtime *Cerner* associates celebrate the anniversary. In a tribute to its roots, *Cerner* donated three picnic tables to Kansas City's Loose Park.

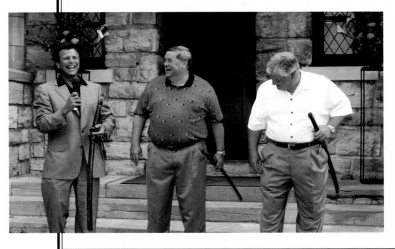

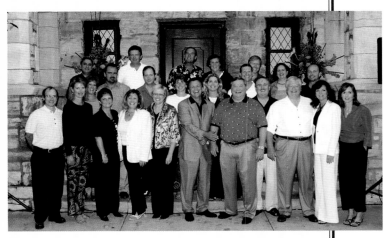

This method saved engineers the valuable time they would have spent troubleshooting every time the system crashed.[33]

The first Millennium conversion was completed in 1997 at Integris Baptist Medical Center, a 508-bed hospital in northwest Oklahoma City. Team directors Bryan Ince and Jeff Townsend managed the conversion with some ideas borrowed from Fred Brooks' classic book *The Mythical Man-Month: Essays on Software Engineering*, published in 1975. One of the concepts that they found particularly helpful was the delegation of an inside and outside man.

"You have an inside guy that you try to keep away from the market, the clients, the salespeople," explained Townsend. "He works directly with the engineers. He does a fair amount of the design of the architecture. Your outside guy needs to be able to do that, but his job is to keep people away from the inside guy."[34]

During the first Millennium conversion, Townsend was the outside man who managed the project and spent a lot of time on site at Integris. Ince was the inside man at *Cerner* headquarters.

Towsend said, "I'm on the phone with him, saying, 'All right, this is code we need to model. Go check up on this team. It doesn't look like their stuff is working.' So it was a dual-headed thing and worked really, really well."[35]

Three HNA Millennium solutions were brought online at Integris: the lab solution *PathNet*®, the Open Clinical Foundation (OCF), and the electronic medical record solution, *PowerChart*®. Approximately 50 engineers worked at Integris around the clock in two 12-hour shifts, and weekly goals were set as they moved toward the go-live deadline in February 1997.

For the most part, the conversion went smoothly due to the architecture's solid design, which prevented major problems such as system crashes. For the implementation team, the most stressful events were the scheduled visits from Patterson, which were designed to help move the process forward. He flew down from time to time, both to provide a morale boost to the team and to keep the schedule on track.

During one visit, when the conversion was nearly complete, Patterson brought a box filled with 500 hats that were embroidered with the text "Integris/*Cerner* First Millennium Conversion, February 1997" to help everyone involved celebrate the conversion.

Townsend and Ince had predicted that the conversion would be completed in February, but toward the end of the month they realized they would need a little more time. Hospital clinicians and administrators said they, too, needed another week, and Townsend agreed that scheduling extra time was the right thing to do. That would move the go-live date into March, leading Townsend to wonder what he should do with the 500 "February" hats. He considered getting the team together at a bar one night to pull out the stitching, but eventually he came up with a better idea.

"If I handed out those hats with the wrong date, they were going to make fun of me," he said. "So we ended up deciding we were going to do a mock conversion just to do a dry run. We'd run it for four hours and see how [everything] would go. If you'd get on the system and practice and try to do your work for an hour, you'd earn a hat." They ran the test in February, and all went well. "It saved the day," said Townsend. "The client loved the hats, and I didn't have the problem of missing the thing by a month."[36]

Once the new architecture went live in March 1997, Ince stayed onsite with a few other team members to make sure everything was running smoothly. His long history of converting *Cerner* solutions had led him to expect a minor problem here or there, but this time, much to the hospital staff's amusement, he didn't have much to do.

"I would walk the floors just to make sure everything was okay, and the nurses would make fun of me," Ince said. "There weren't any problems, and I kept walking around looking for problems. They'd see me coming and start laughing."[37]

The second Millennium conversion, also in 1997, took place at Hermann Memorial Hospital in Houston, Texas. As in Oklahoma City, the team brought OCF, *PathNet*®, and *PowerChart*® to the large metropolitan hospital.

Highs and Lows: A Company in Transition

With two alpha sites successfully converted, *Cerner* could support its sales and marketing efforts with proof positive of Millennium's superior quality. As a result, 187 Millennium solutions were in operation in various facilities by the end of 1998. As Millennium began to make its mark in the industry, the company recovered some of its investment with

A New Logo for a New Era

In 2001, *CERNER* UNVEILED A NEW COMpany logo that was similar to the original but "more streamlined, powerful and contemporary in design," according to Vicki Carlew, vice president of marketing. The new three-part image represents three aspects of the company—the partial circular shape is the letter "C" for *Cerner*, the top bar represents the company's knowledge and solutions, and the lower bar is the healthcare industry.[1]

The long-held former logo contained eight lines moving out of the circle, each of a different length. This aspect of the design, which is retained in the lengths of the two bars in the new logo, signified another core aspect of the company.

"We liked something that implied some motion, that implied incompleteness," said cofounder Cliff Illig of the first logo. "The stylized C, the circle with the lines coming together and then moving out of the circle, but appearing incomplete by being different lengths [made up] a really neat design that matched how we described the company, how we described where we were going."[2]

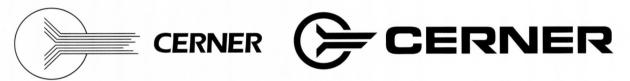

a 35 percent increase in revenues in 1998 to a record $330.9 million, a net earnings increase of 56 percent to $23.7 million, and increased earnings per share of 56 percent to $.70 per share.[38]

In spite of the earnings increase, the value of *Cerner* stock fell to a nearly five-year low in the spring of 1999. On March 17, the stock price dropped to $12.75.[39] Two major factors led to this decline: not enough new enterprise-wide client sales in the latter half of 1998 and growing concern within the healthcare industry about the potential for computer problems at the turn of the century to the year 2000.

The company was "extremely disappointed with *Cerner*'s current shareholder value" in early 1999, and stated that the value did not reflect HNA Millennium and *Cerner*'s standing as an industry leader. The low stock value "leads us to believe we have not been successful in communicating *Cerner*'s basic core strategies and our relative marketplace position," the company told shareholders in the 1998 annual report. "It is crucial that you understand that the investments we have made together in HNA Millennium uniquely position *Cerner* to transform healthcare, and we expect them to eventually transform *Cerner*'s shareholder value."[40]

Stock analysts recognized that many healthcare organizations postponed investing in large-scale IT systems as the threat of Y2K problems heated up in late 1998 and into 1999.[41] Instead, they spent money on electronic systems to help them prepare for Y2K disaster survival.

"We believe that Y2K continues to have an impact on the timing of purchasing decisions within our industry," Patterson said in April 1999. "Some buyers are approaching the marketplace with a great amount of caution, creating a longer decision process, and other potential buyers have temporarily left the marketplace until they complete their Y2K projects."[42]

The Y2K Fiasco

Concerns over Y2K built slowly but powerfully throughout every industry, from banking to healthcare. The potential problems concerned two little digits. In computer systems that had not prepared for the century change to 2000, an entry of "2000" would result in saving the digits "00," and the date would appear as "1900." The ensuing chaos that this glitch was expected to bring to schedules, appointments, insurance claims, and other date-driven entries

Cerner, however, had already prepared its solutions for year 2000 dating in the design of its *Classic* architecture and, subsequently, in HNA Millennium solutions. As early as Classic V300, dates had been stored with a century indicator, eliminating the chance for error with the arrival of 2000.[43] The century indicator became part of *PathNet®*, as the solution was designed to handle the prospect of a 100-year-old person's lab records.

"In the lab," Townsend explained, "you get your blood levels compared to reference ranges, and your reference ranges are sex- and age-sensitive. So, since we had to deal with a 100-year-old patient from day one, that [had to be] figured in when the company started."[44]

In early March 1999, the special U.S. Senate committee that oversaw Y2K preparedness issued a warning about healthcare's lack of readiness for the turn of the century. In a report, Senator Robert F. Bennett, chairman of the Special Committee on the Year 2000 Technology Problem, criticized medical organizations for lagging behind other industries in preparing for potential Y2K emergencies. He cited a lack of planning on the part of hospital administrators and a low degree of awareness among doctors. He also identified healthcare as the worst-prepared industry for the Y2K problem. In addition, Bennett singled out the Medicare program as seriously unprepared. He said:

The healthcare industry is large and incredibly fragmented. I don't believe the healthcare industry's lack of preparedness will necessarily mean loss of life, but it could seriously impact care for millions of Americans dependent on prescription drugs and regular medical treatments to stay healthy. And Medicare, the backbone of our nation's healthcare payment system, is in serious trouble. The agency has completed no end-to-end testing of its external and internal payment systems, so we can only hope that Medicare's billion-dollars-a-day in payments to hospitals and caregivers continue to find their way through the high-tech maze.[45]

Even though *Cerner* was confident that its solutions would not be affected, this certainty did not lessen the company's need to deal with the potential crisis as Y2K frenzy rolled throughout the healthcare industry. *Cerner*'s response to the call for more readiness in the sector included the formation of a consulting group that focused entirely on providing Y2K readiness services for *Cerner* clients. Carol Hull, a manager who started as a programmer at *Cerner* in 1987, was selected to start and direct the group.

"We always want clients to be able to simulate as closely as possible the real world," Hull said. "So we spent a lot of time working with clients getting notes set up so we could actually advance the clock and look at how the software was going to behave ... as we rolled past midnight. We relived the year 2000 several times throughout the course of those months."[46]

The consulting group published a *Y2K Readiness Guide* for associates, which outlined the protocols for dealing with possible problems resulting from the transition from December 31, 1999, to the new year. It also issued a Y2K newsletter to keep its clients updated on testing strategies. The company set up a triage support center modeled after a hospital emergency department to run from the first time change—which would affect *Cerner* clients in Australia on December 31 at 7:00 A.M. Central Time—and run throughout the weekend and the next week.

The triage strategy consisted of round-the-clock teams of support experts who were prepared to quickly route problems to the appropriate teams for troubleshooting. In the case of a power outage, an area on the fourth floor of the 2800 building was set up with a power generator and network and phone systems that would allow associates to continue working on client problems.[47]

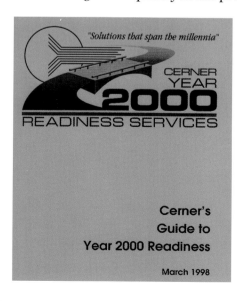

"Solutions that span the millennia"

CERNER YEAR 2000 READINESS SERVICES

Cerner's Guide to Year 2000 Readiness

March 1998

Although *Cerner*'s own solutions were originally designed with a century-naming code, the Y2K consulting group published this readiness guide to help clients prepare for possible computer glitches at the turn of the century.

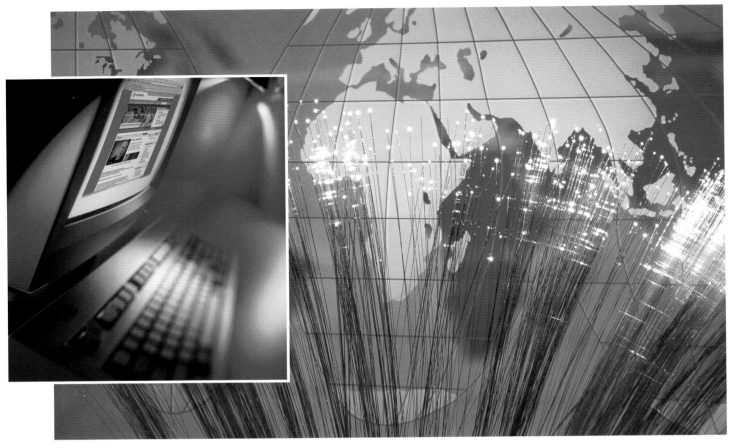

In 2001, *BusinessWeek* named *Cerner* the No. 1 information technology company in the world. That year, the company also made *Fortune*'s list of the "100 Best Companies to Work for in America" and *Forbes*' "Top 200 Best Small Businesses."

The trial runs performed by Hull's consulting group grew into nearly 1,000 "extra projects" for clients, most of which were conducted without charge. *Cerner* clients spent billions putting emergency systems into place and reworking non-*Cerner* components of their medical IT systems to ensure that their patients would not be affected by a technology malfunction.

The carefully prepared triage team had a quiet New Year's Eve. As a result, at 9:00 A.M. on the morning of January 1, 2000, a portion of the on-site teams was allowed to leave in a "partial standdown." The entire emergency operation closed up later that afternoon in a "full standdown." After the new year came and went without a glitch, the

company summed up the Y2K phenomenon as a non-event. Its 1999 annual report stated:

> At midnight, December 31, 1999, the two-digit date field in many legacy computer applications rolled from '99 to '00. Our clients spent billions of dollars preparing for Y2K, an expenditure that generated little incremental value toward improving their capabilities to lower cost, improve quality, or make healthcare delivery safer. The good news is that Y2K is now history.[48]

Early in the new year, Patterson further described the burdens that the Y2K episode had imposed on the entire healthcare industry. In an interview for *The Wall Street Transcript*, Patterson said:

> The Y2K threat instilled uncertainty within all organizations dependent on computers. Y2K clearly had a negative impact on the size of the healthcare information technology marketplace during the last

18 months. Health systems stopped investing in new technology. There were a number of healthcare providers, prospective clients, who decided not to begin new projects. Instead, they expended energy and resources to [upgrade] their current systems. I believe that our entire industry is thankful that Y2K is history.[49]

Cerner 2000 Forms Large-Scale Partnerships

To prepare for HNA Millennium's capabilities in connecting large facilities and communities, *Cerner* launched a business initiative called *Cerner* 2000 in 1995. This program was part of an effort to establish strategic relationships with major health organizations throughout the United States and the world. With these clients, *Cerner* could create models of enterprise-wide efficiency that represented the company's vision for the future of healthcare. The plan also included forming partnerships with companies that provided physician management services, a business known in healthcare as a Management Service Organization (MSO). In these cases, *Cerner* would provide the IT capabilities for such services.

Another component of this vision for the future was a new program to document the benefits of implementing *Cerner*'s solutions and services. With hard data about the way these solutions improve a health organization's finances and level of care, *Cerner* could show prospective clients how the solutions would benefit them.

One of the earliest *Cerner* 2000 alliances was created in 1995 with Health Midwest, the largest health services provider in the Kansas City area. *Cerner* became Health Midwest's exclusive IT partner in this long-term relationship, and the two organizations began working together to build a "new and highly efficient model of care"[50] that exemplified the large-scale, networked vision promised by HNA Millennium.

In January 1996, *Cerner* hired Jack Newman, Jr., a certified public accountant who specialized in healthcare consulting, to direct the *Cerner* 2000 program.[51] Part of Newman's job was to help the company gear its sales force toward forming relationships with large, integrated healthcare organizations like Health Midwest.[52]

"*Cerner* recognizes that as health systems continue to evolve, they will include a broad array of provider/payer components," said Illig when Newman joined the company. "We are committed to being the leader in helping build the key decision-making and knowledge-transfer linkages among these components to enable them to function as a seamless, cost-effective continuum."[53]

While Health Midwest was acquired by the for-profit health system HCA in 2003, the broad business partnership between it and *Cerner* had proven fruitful, particularly in the advancement of *Cerner*'s lab automation services.

Co-Founder Gorup Returns

In 1999, Paul Gorup returned to *Cerner* after a 12-year absence, during which time he had founded a new broadcast radio and TV monitoring company called Broadcast Data Systems (BDS). Launched with two other partners, BDS became the largest commercial system of its kind in the world, monitoring more than 1,100 radio stations and 600 television stations in the United States and Canada. The system detects approximately 120 million occurrences of music and commercial airplay each year and sends this information directly to clients such as Billboard, which then uses the information, among other factors, to create the Top 40 charts.

Although the broadcasting industry was a completely new playing field for Gorup, it provided him with an opportunity to apply his technical expertise to fulfill a well-defined need in the market, just as *Cerner* had done.

"I always say that I'm probably one of the only people to have my picture in *Billboard* magazine and the *College of American Pathology Today*," Gorup said. "My kids thought it was probably the neatest job in the world. 'My Dad knows the Top 40 chart better than anybody else!', they'd say, and they loved listening to our huge CD collection and being around when stars came to the building. So it was a neat job for the kids growing up."[54]

Gorup and his partners sold BDS in 1995, just when *Cerner* was beginning to develop Millennium. Although he stayed in touch and was aware of this new development, he did not come back to the company until 1999. "I needed to decide, sooner or later, what I was going to do when I grew up," he said. "I felt I had one good spurt in my career left, and I always tell people that BDS was fun, but

CERNER HONORS AND AWARDS

2005

- Rockhurst University's Helzberg School of Management and the Kansas City chapter of the Society of Financial Service Professionals
- 2005 Kansas City Business Ethics Award.
- *The Kansas City Star*'s Star 50 list of top metropolitan companies (ranked No. 6).
- *Business 2.0*: Fastest-Growing Technology Companies (ranked No. 43).
- *ComputerWorld* Honors Collection: Medal of Achievement.
- TEPR (Toward Electronic Patient Records) Awards: First Honors for Electronic Health Record Systems for Hospitals.
- *ComputerWorld* and the Storage Networking Industry Association Award to *Cerner*Works for exemplary storage networking solutions.

2004

- Oracle Partner of the Year.
- 2004 Missouri Pro Patria Award presented to employers demonstrating exceptional support for national defense by adopting personnel policies that make it easier for employees to participate in the National Guard and Reserve. The award was created by the National Committee of Employer Support of the Guard and Reserve, an agency within the Office of the Assistant Secretary of Defense for Reserve Affairs.
- KLAS Market Intelligence Leaders: *Cerner Millennium PathNet*®, Most Improved Performance as reported by Healthcare Professionals in 2003.
- No. 1 in 2004 DKWS Securities Vendor Ranking.
- TEPR Awards: First Honors for Electronic Health Record Systems for Hospitals.

- TEPR Awards: Second Honors for Medical Records/Document Imaging Management Systems.
- *Training Magazine*: Top 100 (No. 78).
- American Society for Training & Development, Kansas City: Best Practice in Skills Transformation.

2003

- Five Rights' 2003 Medication Safety Tools. *Cerner*'s CPOE earned the best scores in the report's "high priority" criteria among generally available solutions.
- *The Kansas City Star*'s Star 50 (No. 8).
- *Computer World*: 100 Best Places To Work In IT (No. 31).
- *Kansas City Business Journal*: Top 25 Fastest Growing Companies (No. 19).
- Paragon Facet of Excellence Award.

2002

- 2002 Governor's Achievement Award.
- Business Attraction and Expansion Award.
- *The Kansas City Star*'s Star 50 (No. 41).
- TEPR Awards: Security (Second Honors).
- Woman of Color in Health Sciences and Technology Award: Lori Bunch, vice president of product management.
- 2002 Society of Environmental Graphics Merit Award: *Cerner* Identity Structure.
- 2002 *International Design* magazine's Annual Design Review: *Cerner* Identity Structure.
- American Society for Training & Development, Kansas City: Best Practices Award in Training Through Technological Advances.
- American Society for Training & Development, Kansas City: Exceptional Leadership Award: Rob Campbell, vice president of learning.

2001

- *Fortune* magazine's "100 Best Companies to Work for in America" (No. 56).
- *Ingram's* magazine's Corporate 100 (No. 99).
- *Business Week*'s No. 1 IT company.
- *Kansas City Star*'s Star 50 (No. 4).
- VARBusiness 500 (No. 110).
- Deloitte & Touche Fast 50.
- *Forbes* magazine's Top 200 Best Small Businesses (No. 86).
- Healthcare Informatics Top 100 HIT Companies, based on healthcare IT revenue generated only from IT products and services (No. 7).
- 2001 Young Architects Award: *Cerner* Identity Structure.
- 2001 Kansas City AIA Arts & Craftsmanship Award: *Cerner* Vision Center Portals.

2000

- Deloitte & Touche Fast 50: Kansas/Western Missouri Technology Fast 50 Award.
- *Ingram's* magazine, Best of Business Kansas City: Best Employer Award, Bronze Award.

1999

- *Fortune*'s "100 Best Companies to Work for in America."
- Paragon Award for Excellence in Human Resources Practices.
- *Ingram's* magazine, Best of Business Kansas City: Best Employer Award, Bronze Award.

1995

- Professional Secretaries International, Missouri Division: Recognition Plus Program.
- *Ingram's* magazine: Salute One of the Corporate Report 100, Kansas City's Fastest Growing Companies.

1994

- *BusinessWeek*: One of the 100 Best Small Corporations.
- Professional Secretaries International Missouri Division: Recognition of Outstanding Performance.

1993

- Clay County Economic Development Council: 1993 Keystone Award.
- *Ingram's* magazine: Salute One of the Corporate Report 100, Kansas City's Fastest Growing Companies.

1991

- Hi-Tech Entrepreneurs, Western Missouri/Kansas: Entrepreneurs of the Year.

1990

- *Forbes*: The 200 Best Small Companies in America.

1988

- *BusinessWeek*: One of the 100 Best Small Corporations.
- *Inc.* magazine: Fastest Growing Small Public Companies.
- Corporate Report 100: Kansas City's Fastest Growing Companies.
- The Chamber of Commerce for Greater Kansas City: Small Business of the Year Award.

1987

- *Inc.* magazine: Fastest Growing Small Public Companies.[1]

making Madonna a lot of money didn't make you feel really good at night. *Cerner* always made you feel good at night."[55]

Upon his return, Gorup was named vice president of application data services, a position in which he helped develop *Cerner*'s Millennium solutions for the Web. He also spearheaded the creation of new data centers at *Cerner* headquarters and in Lee's Summit, Missouri. In 2002, he became president of *Cerner*'s newest organization, Knowledge and Discovery, which develops new Millennium solutions.

"When I came back, [I realized] distance makes the heart fonder," Gorup said. "I think all of us appreciate a lot more where we had been, what we have done." Gorup is pleased to be working with his former partners again and is readjusting to Patterson's style of continuously looking for inroads to growth. "It's nice to have somebody that sits back and looks at that and can challenge you. I think I complement him very well in that he can put a stake in the ground, and I can get there fairly fast, fairly directly."[56]

9/11 Tragedy Strikes
During Health Conference

Another defining moment for the company came, as it did for many individuals and corporations around the world, with the terrorist attacks of September 11, 2001. That year, *Cerner*'s annual health conference was scheduled for September 9 through 12 in Bartle Hall, one of the large exhibition spaces at the Kansas City Convention Center. With approximately 2,000 guests and 1,000 *Cerner* associates attending and manning the exhibits, the first two days and nights of the convention went smoothly.

On the morning of September 11, keynote speaker Matt Ridley was on stage in the Bartle Hall auditorium talking about his book, *Genome: The Autobiography of a Species in 23 Chapters*, with slides projected on two large screens behind him. As soon as *Cerner* executives heard the news about the first attack on the World Trade Center in New York City, they projected CNN onto one of the screens. As word spread, associates and guests thronged into the 3,000-seat auditorium to watch the events unfold. The big question for the company was, "Do we continue the conference or shut down?"

Then-Chief People Officer Stan Sword was one of the executives on the scene that morning who helped decide how to proceed. "What do you do?" he said. "You don't want to overreact, but you don't really know what's going on yet."[57] Sword recalled the conflicting images in the auditorium, where Ridley's slides about the future of scientific discovery clashed with CNN reports of death and destruction.

"On the one hand," Sword said, "you've got the ability for man to create new science and have a better understanding of the basic building blocks of life, and [a discussion of] what we are going to do with that as a society. So man's ability to create was on one screen, and on the other was man's ability to destroy. It was just incredibly striking, the contrast."[58]

Associates set up television sets in the hallways so that all the conference attendees could stay informed. Other healthcare IT companies who were also holding events at the time did not take the same approach. "We happened to have a couple of competitors that had their conference at the same time," Townsend said. "They chose not to show the stuff. So we immediately filled the halls with TVs. Everywhere you went, it was on."[59]

Immediately after the attacks, Walt Foultz, *Cerner*'s chief security officer at the time, contacted the FBI and began planning evacuation procedures to get the thousands of guests and associates out of Bartle Hall if needed. Throughout that morning, no one knew if the terrorists would strike other targets—such as a major metropolitan area like Kansas City.

Another issue was that key officials from facilities close to "ground zero" were attending the conference, such as the CEOs of healthcare organizations in New York, Washington, D.C., and Boston. "Our first instincts were that we need to get those people home," Sword said.[60] Knowing that the airlines would be shut down, *Cerner* contacted the bus company that provided shuttle service between the hotels and the convention center during the conference and hired it to drive convention guests to the major East Coast cities and elsewhere.

"We put a *Cerner* associate on each bus and made sure they had a corporate calling card and cell phones and batteries and a credit card and said, 'now your job is to make sure these people get home safely,'" Sword said. "Within an hour of the tower being hit, we had plans in place, stations set up, to care for the people."[61]

Associates handed over their cars to conference guests or invited them to stay in their homes until transportation could be arranged, as many had already checked out of their hotels that morning with plans to leave the conference on the 11th. Associates went home to make box lunches and cookies for their clients to take on the bus or in a car for their road trips home. "I think it was a very memorable event, especially for clients and associates that were in from all over the world," Townsend said. "You had our folks riding on buses with our clients for 14 hours or whatever, headed to the East Coast."[62]

The many crises of that historic day included a conference guest who needed to get to Los Angeles after her father suddenly became critically ill. *Cerner* hired a limousine and two drivers to take her back to Los Angeles, driving straight through so that she could see her father before he died.

Another now-legendary event occurred on the bus taking guests back home to New Jersey, New York, and Connecticut. Jay Kim, a *Cerner* client executive who had been with the company for just five months, was one of the associates designated to accompany the 40 passengers on the bus. As the bus headed down the interstate highway through Pennsylvania at about 3 A.M., Kim was awakened by the sound of scraping. He quickly discovered that the bus had tipped to one side and was scraping against the metal guard rail along the side of the road. Kim jumped over the sleeping passenger next to him and ran to the front of the bus.

Tom Kemp, chief information officer at New York Hospital Medical Center in Queens was seated just behind the driver and was also woken by the scraping sound. Both men found the driver slumped in his seat, unconscious. Kemp grabbed the wheel, and he and Kim managed to get the driver's foot off the accelerator and stop the bus. They rushed the driver outside onto the ground and administered CPR, but he had suffered a massive heart attack, and they were unable to resuscitate him. Their fast actions did, however, save the lives of the 40 passengers on the bus.

The new driver, who would take the wheel on the next leg of the trip, had known the deceased driver for several years. One of the passengers said, "When Roger had to proceed driving after learning of his friend's death, Jay didn't sit down in his chair, he sat on the floor next to Roger. He joined Roger at the front of the bus, conversed with him, kept the conversation

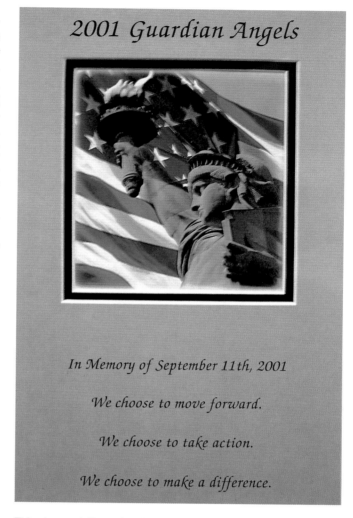

2001 Guardian Angels

In Memory of September 11th, 2001

We choose to move forward.

We choose to take action.

We choose to make a difference.

This plaque at *Cerner* headquarters honors the associates who went above and beyond the call of duty in helping health conference attendees to return home safely after the 9/11 terrorist attacks. *(Photo of plaque by Antonia Felix.)*

light, and made sure Roger was able to drive us to meet the new driver.... He was remarkable."[63]

The "treat others as you would like to be treated" aspect of *Cerner* culture that the founders had learned from Ewing Kauffman was clearly put into practice during the 9/11 crisis. Many associates were recognized as "guardian angels" for the help they provided clients at that time, and a photo of approximately 150 associates who went above and beyond the call of duty hangs on the wall of the 2800 building.

"You can't demand people to give of themselves the way people gave, but they did it because they knew it was the right thing to do and wanted to do it and wanted to help," Sword said. "It's something that really made me proud."[64]

The Bet Pays Off

After the Y2K jitters had passed, HNA Millennium quickly began providing the company with a return on its investment, and the first conversions provided support for *Cerner*'s greatly expanded sales force. At the end of 2000, Millennium solutions were operating in 125 organizations throughout the world, and revenues jumped 19 percent over the previous year.[65]

In 2001, another record year, 40 percent of the company's sales went to clients who had never before purchased *Cerner* solutions. That year, revenues increased 35 percent over the previous year.[66] Revenue continued to increase in 2002, climbing 39 percent over 2001 to $780 million.[67]

"We have grown the top line every single year in our 23-year history," the 2002 annual report stated. "Clearly growth is part of our culture."[68]

Although revenue increased overall in 2003, a first-quarter shortfall had a negative ripple effect, and by the end of the year, the increase over 2002 was only 8 percent. The shortfall raised flags and prompted the company to investigate whether it was heading for a downward shift within the marketplace. The company's review did not find any evidence of such a trend, however, and client bookings increased in each of the next three quarters of the year.

But the unexpected first-quarter performance did precipitate a series of shareholder lawsuits, which were later dismissed. On April 3, the company announced that it was lowering its first-quarter forecasts for earnings and revenue due to "a change in the competitive environment," Patterson said in a news release. He added that "more challenging economics for healthcare provider organizations resulted in us losing some deals we expected to win and some deals being pushed out of the quarter."[69]

Cerner's stock price fell from $32.09 on April 2 to $18.55 on April 3 following the announcement, a drop of 43 percent.[70]

Immediately, three shareholder groups filed lawsuits, claiming that *Cerner* had committed securities fraud by not accurately reporting its position in the market. The company attributed the lawsuits to a common yet regrettable practice of the times.

"The lawsuits are a reflection of the unfortunate litigious environment that we live in," said Randy Sims, *Cerner*'s chief legal officer.[71] The annual report released in early 2004 echoed Sims' explanation. It stated:

Wall Street is conditioned to act very quickly to any quarterly results that vary from expectations, and after meeting or exceeding their consensus estimates for 13 quarters in a row, our single miss cut the stock price nearly in half to $16.50. There is a segment of the legal system in this country that promotes the filing of class-action lawsuits against companies in such circumstances, and Cerner was no exception. We strongly believe the lawsuit filed against Cerner is without merit, and we are vigorously defending it.[72]

By the end of 2003, the stock price rebounded to $37.85, up 21 percent from the end of 2002,[73] demonstrating that the scare at the beginning of the year did not signal a downturn for the company. The courts later upheld *Cerner*'s motion to dismiss and the class action lawsuits were discarded in June 2004.

Revenues continued to increase in the first three quarters of 2004, and new bookings in the first quarter of 2004 were up 43 percent over the same period in 2003.[74] New bookings in the second quarter increased by 19 percent compared to the same quarter in 2003, and new bookings in the third quarter were up 6 percent from the third quarter of the previous year. By the end of 2004, *Cerner*'s Millennium solutions were online at 749 facilities worldwide.[75]

When *Cerner* announced its fourth-quarter and full-year 2004 results on February 3, 2005, its stock price had climbed to $50.44 a share. The day after the announcement, the price climbed again to $52.67 as a result of the year's excellent performance. Full-year earnings per share were $1.73, a 47 percent increase over 2003. The company reported record operating cash flow of $168.3 million for the year and—after deducting capital expenditures and capitalized software—a record $53 million of free cash flow. In addition, a record 1,079 Millennium conversions took place in 2004.[76]

The analysts' reports that appeared after this announcement highlighted *Cerner*'s leading role in the industry and predicted continued growth and success.

Andrew Weinberger of Bear Stearns & Company wrote, "Twenty-nine percent of bookings dollars came from new customers ... which is near the low end of CERN's historical 25 percent–40 percent (but well above any other competitor in the industry), illustrating that CERN remains the clear clinical IT leader."[77]

Reporting for the firm WR Hambrecht, Sean Wieland wrote, "We believe CERN is a core holding in the HCIT space because of its market leadership position, breadth and depth of its product portfolio, and strong earnings growth."[78]

Ryan Stewart at Piper Jaffray noted the role that the company's diabetes PHR initiative played in the industry: "We view CERN's juvenile diabetes program as directionally supporting the role HCIT will likely play in an eventual information-driven healthcare system."[79]

Jim Kumpel of Friedman, Billings, Ramsey & Company reinforced this view of *Cerner* as a present and future leader. "We continue to believe that the positive developments in Washington surrounding the need for healthcare IT investments and clinical systems are bullish for CERN's business long term," he wrote.[80]

Glen Santangelo of Jefferies & Company acknowledged *Cerner*'s innovative role in the industry and concluded that its long history of success would continue.

"In our view, *Cerner* had the vision to create a unified technology platform at a time when its competitors were still selling modular, best-of-breed solutions, and has benefited from this decision, as evidenced by strong bookings, revenue, and earnings growth over the past several years," Santangelo wrote. "We believe potential margin expansion over the next few years represents a significant opportunity for *Cerner*, as it is poised to leverage previous invest-

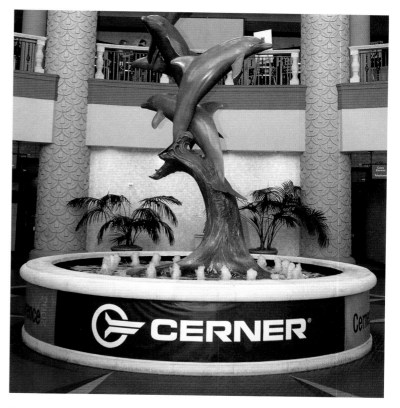

The redesigned *Cerner* logo received plenty of exposure at the 2005 *Cerner* Health Conference in Orlando, Florida.

ments. We believe the company's strategic vision and solid execution have yielded evident returns in strong sales, earnings, and bookings growth over the past several years and should position the company for future success."[81]

In December 2005, the board of directors announced a 2-for-1 stock split of the company's common stock, increasing the common shares issued and outstanding from approximately 38.4 million to 76.8 million. With stocks trading as high as $98 in 2005, *Cerner*'s market value has continued to climb.

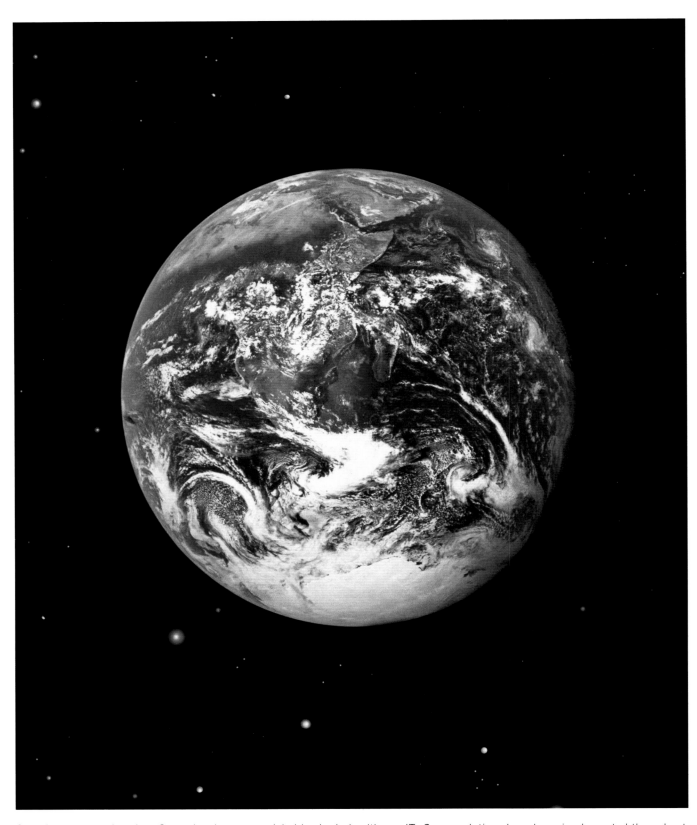

Over the past two decades, *Cerner* has become a global leader in healthcare IT. *Cerner* solutions have been implemented throughout Europe, Asia, Australia, and the Middle East.

CHAPTER SEVEN

A SOLID BASE GROWS GLOBALLY

We think our future growth will depend on our success in the global markets. The world is a big place, and 55 percent of all world healthcare IT spend[ing] is outside the U.S. So we want to be positioned to be a player there, and we're working hard to do that.

—Trace Devanny, *Cerner* president[1]

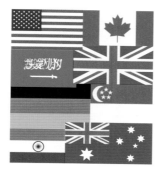

ERNER'S DOMESTIC SUCCESS with the *PathNet*® laboratory solution and other HNA Classic solutions in the 1980s led to an ambitious international strategy in the 1990s. The company expanded into several international locations before exploding onto the global scene with the turn of the millennium. Most notably, in 2003 *Cerner* began pursuing its first government partnership in response to an effort by England's National Health Service to automate that nation's healthcare system.

Cerner was eventually awarded what may have been the most strategic assignment—the electronic appointment booking system for the entire country—and the company treated the experience as an invaluable investment in the future. It later also won the coveted opportunity to become the healthcare IT solution provider for the entire southern region of England. This included the challenge of converting and connecting healthcare facilities throughout the region.

At the start of the new century, *Cerner* continued to secure contracts with additional clients around the world, strengthening the company's position as a global leader in healthcare IT.

Raising Standards Throughout the World

Cerner's first forays into the global market occurred in 1985 when it converted *PathNet*® in

Canada and in 1986 when it entered into a licensing deal with McDonnell Douglas for *PathNet*® sales in the United Kingdom. *Cerner* increased its presence in the United Kingdom in 1991 by forming *Cerner* Limited and assuming the *PathNet*® service relationship that McDonnell Douglas had initiated with 16 hospitals in England. *Cerner* entered into these client relationships in conjunction with the Northwest Thames Regional Health Authority in London, and from its new London office began formulating a strategy to increase sales throughout that country.[2]

One extensive marketing program was targeted at Scotland, where healthcare administrators were actively seeking electronic solutions. In 1992, Health Care International, Ltd., in Clydebank, Scotland, agreed to convert to an entire suite of *Cerner* solutions. The following year, it added *Cerner* solutions in the lab, radiology, and pharmacy departments, and were automating the patient record, registration, clinical ordering and scheduling, decision support, and patient discharge protocols.[3]

Cerner's active international effort in the early 1990s was not limited to Europe. The company had established an office in Australia in 1991, the same

---

Cerner's international efforts established crucial partnerships for the company all over the world.

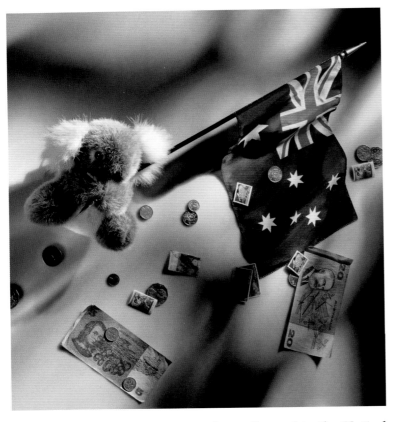

year that *Cerner* Limited was formed in the United Kingdom. The new subsidiary, *Cerner* Corporation Pty. Limited, in Sydney, was initiated by a contract with the state of New South Wales to install and support *PathNet®* in two hospitals. These facilities were the pilot sites for a government contract with the potential to reach the remaining 60 hospitals operated by the New South Wales Health Department.[4] In 1992, the London and Sydney offices were bustling with activity, with 20 full-time associates working in each office.

Cerner entered the Asian market with *PathNet®* sales to the Singapore Public Health system in 1991. These conversions included the National Healthcare Group in the west and were a precursor to what would become a major *Cerner* presence in that part of the world.[5]

At the same time, *Cerner* made its first entrée into the Middle East when it agreed to convert its lab solution at the Riyadh Armed Forces Hospital in Riyadh, Saudi Arabia. Riyadh, the capital city, had a population of more than 2 million in 1991 and has been growing by nearly 8 percent a year ever since.[6] The military hospital conversions were the product

of *Cerner*'s joint partnership with the El Seif Health Care Group, the largest healthcare organization in Saudi Arabia. By 1996, 21 *Cerner* associates were at work in Saudi Arabia, and the joint partnership had succeeded in implementing *Cerner* solutions at five sites in Saudi Arabia and one in the United Arab Emirates.

Back in Europe, *Cerner* began targeting German healthcare companies in 1992, and the following

Left: The *Cerner* Corporation Pty. Ltd. subsidiary was established in Sydney, Australia, in 1991, when the company contracted with the state of New South Wales to install and support *PathNet®* in two hospitals.

Below: *Cerner*'s laboratory solution, *PathNet®*, was translated into German in 1993 for a conversion at the Klinikum Chemnitz hospital.

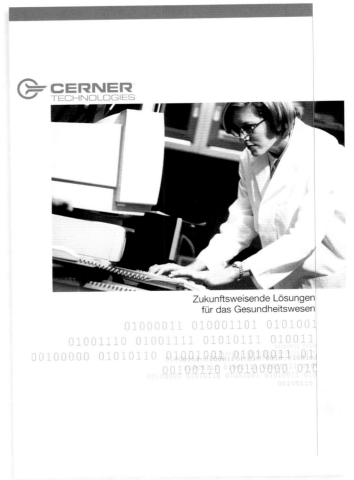

SIMPLIFYING GERMAN HEALTHCARE

IN 1996, *CERNER* BECAME INVOLVED with Klinikum Chemnitz, one of Germany's largest hospitals with 1,850 beds. Situated in five networked locations within the city of Chemnitz, the hospital provides care for more than 65,000 inpatients and 160,000 outpatients every year.

"To be able to ensure that patients are given the very best of treatment in a hospital this size, all information on the patient must be available at all times and in all places," said Dr. Olaf Schlimpert, head of healthcare IT at Klinikum Chemnitz. "We went for *Cerner* because the system meets all of our transparency and scalability requirements."[1]

As the German health system faced challenges in overcoming budgetary constraints, local hospitals strove to become more economically viable and efficient. The integrated architecture and extensive functionality of *Cerner* solutions provided Klinikum Chemnitz the opportunity to streamline its clinical information system (CIS).

A decade later, *Cerner* Millennium runs on almost all PCs used in Klinikum Chemnitz for medical purposes, with over 2,000 users utilizing the system.

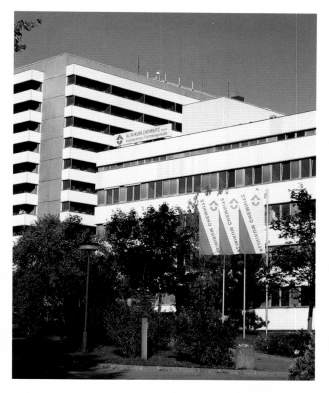

Germany's Klinikum Chemnitz Hospital is equipped with *Cerner*'s state-of-the-art healthcare IT systems.

year *PathNet*® was translated into German for the first time for a conversion at the Klinikum Chemnitz.[7] This 1,850-bed hospital, located in the city of Chemnitz about 160 miles south of Berlin, soon added German-language Classic solutions for radiology and blood bank, which created a hospital-wide paperless order- and result-entry system. Chemnitz continued to build its IT capabilities when *Cerner*'s new architecture was introduced, converting to HNA Millennium solutions such as *PowerChart*®.[8]

The most ambitious conversion in *Cerner*'s history—and the first nationwide healthcare IT system in the world—went online in England in 2004. The previous year, *Cerner* was among a number of companies vying for the National Health Service's (NHS) massive procurement of IT systems to automate and connect healthcare facilities across the nation. The NHS sought an electronic scheduling/booking system for the entire country, plus sophisticated IT systems to automate hospitals and clinics. England had been divided into five regions for the procurement, which would require five Local Service Providers (LSPs), or IT contractors, to convert and maintain the new medical IT solutions. Each region represented an extremely lucrative opportunity.

"In many ways, it was historic what England attempted to do and is attempting to do," said David Sides, managing director of *Cerner* Ltd. "It is the

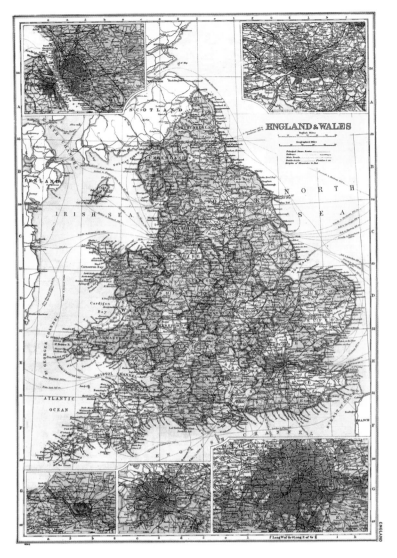

Cerner made its first inroads into the United Kingdom with sales of its automated healthcare solutions in England and Scotland. By 2004, its Choose and Book electronic booking solution was being implemented in several locations. *(Map courtesy of Your Old Books & Maps.)*

largest IT project procurement by far anywhere in the world. Automating, electronically delivering care across 50 million people was absolutely spot-on the right thing to do."[9]

Cerner partnered with a European IT company called SchlumbergerSema (now Atos Origin) in its effort to win some of the contracts. Schlumberger-

Sema had won other major contracts in England—including a system for the national railway service—and *Cerner* hoped to benefit from the other company's experience in delivering IT in England and its knowledge of the nation's infrastructure.[10]

The NHS demanded rigorous proof of solution (POS) exercises from each IT company to help it determine who would win the contracts. In running through these exercises, *Cerner* discovered that its new Millennium architecture was extraordinarily scalable and could deliver the speed necessary for the large, industrial-strength scale of a nationwide system. Never before in history had such a massive test been performed on an automated system, and *Cerner* demonstrated that Millennium could process four electronic bookings a second, utilizing a database with 2.7 billion rows/1.2 terabytes of data.[11] *Cerner*'s test run outperformed NHS requirements at every level, and results included the following highlights:

- Completed project nearly two weeks early;
- Met all Service Level Agreements (SLAs) at 100 percent load, as well as SLAs at 150 percent workload;
- Served 962 active Web users;
- Served 1,525 active Win32 users;
- Performed 79,274 Interface transactions an hour (22 per second);
- Performed 13,987 bookings an hour (four per second);
- Performed 97,550 Web transactions an hour (27 per second);
- Moved $5 million in IBM equipment into the test lab within two weeks;
- Met all service levels at the 150 percent load, which was not a requirement; *Cerner* only had to prove that it could run above 100 percent peak volume load;
- Ran an additional test to determine when actual saturation would occur; system ran up to almost 190 percent before it fully consumed the CPU on the back end application server; *Cerner* did not identify any bottlenecks in the architecture, and increased volume could have been processed with additional hardware.[12]

The POS tests also gave the company an opportunity to build upon its ideas for community-wide

IT systems, an integral part of the company vision. The 2003 annual report stated, "In contemplating healthcare delivery for a nation, we advanced our understanding of our proprietary community model for health and how to apply it to large populations."[13]

When England announced the winners of the contracts in 2004, *Cerner* was disappointed to learn that it had only been granted the scheduling component, the national electronic booking service. From a financial perspective, this was the smallest of the $10 billion in contracts awarded, but it was the first system that would be implemented.[14]

Cerner Chief of Staff Jeff Townsend, who participated in the negotiating process of the contract, worked on a 24-hour schedule in September 2004. "The one contract that we won, eBookings—now called Choose & Book—was a 'round-the-clock negotiating session," he said. "The big commit that we made (in the middle of the night) was that we would prove in 90 days that our solution could scale to meet the volume requirements equivalent to year-two usage, or they could opt out. This was the beginning of changing our thinking about applying our solutions to populations. It was memorable because the contracting session went until 4 A.M. with us toasting champagne."[15]

Cerner's Jon Doolittle, who worked on the NHS procurement for seven months as a market intelligence executive, believed *Cerner* won the contract because it would be the first test of Prime Minister Tony Blair's new healthcare IT plan for his country. "I think that we won [Choose and Book] because it was going to be first, that we clearly had the most mature application," Doolittle said. "We demonstrated that we could do what they needed done, and they didn't want to kick off this whole national program with a lemon."[16]

The electronic booking system, which *Cerner* converted throughout England in August 2004, was designed to help solve one of the biggest problems that plagued England's healthcare system—long waiting lists. The wait for an appointment was extremely long, and in cases of elective surgery, people often had to wait a full year to get a procedure performed. The goal of the new system was to drastically reduce the waiting time for appointments and procedures.

Reflecting on the NHS contract award, Townsend recognized many positives even though the company was initially awarded only one contract. "It changed the way we looked at our marketplace and our solutions," he said. "It spawned [new] efforts. While we didn't walk away with a large amount of business in England, competing for that business forced us to evaluate our delivery, availability, and how an entire region (population or country) could be deployed as quickly and cost effectively as possible."[17]

The lessons learned in England helped *Cerner* continue to shape its vision of large-scale community and regional IT systems. John Kuckelman, vice president of engineering, stated that one of the company's biggest challenges was "being able to have a database that holds a country's worth of medical records, a database that [is] 99.99 percent reliable. This database must have very little down time, if any at all, over the course of the year. It just has to be super, super-reliable."[18]

This was a very different challenge than the database needs of a bank, for example, as Kuckelman explained: "At Bank of America, every Saturday afternoon at noon, they take that database down. As long as they have it back up by Monday morning, it's not a big deal. The number of people, I think, in the world trying to keep systems running perpetually, you could count on two hands probably. A lot of my time has been focused on how to deliver Millennium more reliably, with higher quality, making our clients' experience more robust and more like you're going to go in and it's going to work the first time, and there are not going to be any surprises."[19]

Marc Naughton, senior vice president and chief financial officer, added that the companies who did originally win the contracts in England had a formidable challenge ahead. "We thought we could do it, but we knew it was going to be very hard," he said. "Some of the people that won, I think, are just now beginning to understand that it's going to be really be hard to deliver. In our mind, winning the bookings contract ... could set us up to perhaps step into the shoes of some of the others if they are not successful."[20]

These reflections proved invaluable as *Cerner* continued to bid for contracts on additional services in England, never diminishing its determination to participate in the country's historic healthcare reform. Throughout these processes, *Cerner* formed a partnership with Fujitsu and worked hard to communicate an accurate appraisal of *Cerner*'s capabilities.

This strategy paid off as *Cerner* eventually supplanted its competitor, IDX Systems Corporation, to win the lucrative subcontract of solution provider for the southern region. The resulting deal for *Cerner* and Fujitsu included 142 hospitals and seven strategic health authorities, according to David Sides, managing director of *Cerner* Limited in the United Kingdom.[21] The southern region represents the largest cluster in terms of population and number of deployments.

"What *Cerner* has been doing for coming up on 26 years now is proving that we have these solutions based on a unified architecture that can scale across large hospitals and health systems throughout the U.S.," said Justin Scott, senior manager of marketing. "That scalability has really been proven and tested by the engagement in England with the National Health Service, first with the Choose & Book system and now with the southern cluster of England."[22]

Referring to the extensive scope of the NHS reform, Townsend predicted, "I think that this trend of deploying systems at a wide-scale geographic level or a national level will continue to increase in the coming years."[23]

Cerner gained another foothold in the European market when it acquired the German company Image

Devices in 2002. The two companies had previously formed a partnership in 1999 to develop the *Cerner ProVision*™ picture archiving and communication system (PACS). This solution stores and retrieves digital images, such as MRI and CT scans, to make them electronically accessible to every segment of a healthcare organization.

The new company, Image Devices, a *Cerner* company, retained all of its associates and remained in its original offices in Aachen and Idstein, Germany. With this purchase, *Cerner* gained 80 clients that were using Image Devices' solutions throughout Germany, Switzerland, and Austria.

"Medical images are an integral part of the patient's electronic medical record," said Devanny in a press release about the acquisition. "Bringing Image Devices into *Cerner* will help us to improve our electronic medical record capabilities. In addition, the acquisition will significantly increase our presence in Europe, giving us new clients to which we can introduce *Cerner* solutions."[24]

In 2004, *Cerner* enhanced its ability to develop its software on a 24-hour basis when it opened an office in Bangalore, India. While associates in Kansas City wrote code during the day, software engineers in India ran tests on the software overnight.

"The biggest improvement I can make in how *Cerner* operates is to find a straightforward way of being a 24-hour operation," Patterson said. "And the easiest way to do that is to put a piece of *Cerner* around software development that is 12 hours away from Kansas City."[25]

Patterson commented that the round-the-clock process launched by *Cerner* India allowed the company to expand its development of Intellectual Property (IP).

"During 2004, we successfully extended our IP organization globally by launching *Cerner* India and establishing a portion of the software development cycle (certification) in this part of *Cerner*," he told associates. "This move promises to greatly expand our capabilities by shortening the development cycle by taking advantage of time zone differences. For decades, the sun has never set on our solutions running in healthcare. Now, the sun never sets on our IP development."[26]

When Jeanne Patterson ran as a Republican for a U.S. House of Representatives seat in 2004, her opponent, Democrat and former Kansas City

The *Cerner ProVision*™ picture archiving and communication system (PACS) was developed in 1999 by *Cerner* and Image Devices, a German company acquired by *Cerner* in 2002. PACS has simplified electronic access to digital healthcare images.

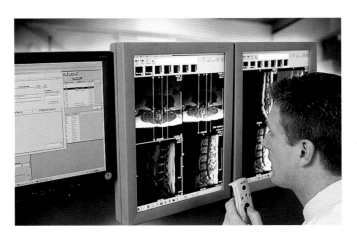

mayor Emanuel Cleaver, attacked Patterson for being affiliated with an "immoral" company that outsourced jobs to India while people in Kansas City looked for work.

Cliff Illig responded through an editorial, asking, for example, why a company that employed more than 3,500 workers in the Kansas City area, had a payroll of more than $250 million, and added local jobs every week, had become the villain in a political race.[27] Patterson eventually lost the Congressional race by a narrow margin. *Cerner*'s Kansas City associate headcount has since grown to more than 4,300.

Although outsourcing to India became a hot-button issue for many American companies in 2003 and 2004—especially in the customer service area—global expansion of sales is a reality for many types of American businesses, and foreign markets are expected to play a very important part in *Cerner*'s future. The company recognizes that its solutions are suitable everywhere because they were designed around the core issue of every healthcare system—the person.

As early as 1992, the annual report described its now-Classic architecture as ready for the future of healthcare in this regard. "There is one constant, one absolute, one focus of healthcare wherever in the world you go: The Patient. And, since *Cerner*'s Healthcare Network Architecture (HNA) is focused on the processes surrounding the patient, our vision is just as applicable throughout the world as it is in the United States."[28]

With *Cerner*'s electronic bookings system in England showing the world the strength of Millennium, the company is poised to continue to expand its presence around the world. The global marketplace is crucial to the company's future suc-

cess, according to Doug Krebs, President of *Cerner* Global Organization.

"When you look at the macro-level economics, well over half of the expenditures today and for the foreseeable future come out of the non-U.S. markets," he explained. "So we don't really have a choice but to grow on a global basis if we're going to continue to grow as we've enjoyed our growth to now."[29]

Devanny voiced the same intent to expand *Cerner*'s global presence. "We think our future growth will depend on our success in the global markets," he said. "The world is a big place, and 55 percent of all world healthcare IT spend[ing] is outside the U.S. So we want to be positioned to be a player there, and we're working hard to do that."[30]

Vice President Mike Breedlove has been with *Cerner* since 1983 and has born witness to enormous expansion. Yet he asserted that the overall growth of the company has not interfered with most of its core elements.

"The dedication and passion of associates to making a difference has not changed in relation to *Cerner*'s size," Breedlove said. "The challenge that we have as an organization is to take the newest college hires and instill in them that same passion, that they can make a difference. I think overall we've done a very good job of that."[31]

According to Breedlove, with *Cerner*'s global growth comes the opportunity to develop the company's architecture up to the next level. He said, "We've proven now that we can do it, handling not just individual or aggregated healthcare institutions, but actually handling the health economy of countries and states. We've proven it now since we've been successful in the U.K. We are serving fifty million people there and it's only just begun."[32]

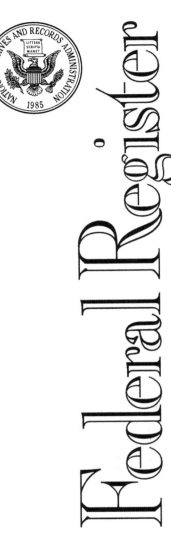

Friday,
April 30, 2004

Part VII

The President

**Executive Order 13335—Incentives for the
Use of Health Information Technology
and Establishing the Position of the
National Health Information Technology
Coordinator**

The prominent role of IT in modern healthcare was highlighted when President George W. Bush created the position of the National Health Information Technology Coordinator in 2004. *(Reprinted with the permission of the Office of the Federal Register.)*

CHAPTER EIGHT

DESIGNS ON THE FUTURE

An important part of Cerner's *future is to make sure that we continue to innovate. There's never a dull moment here. CEO Neal Patterson is as engaged and intense today as he was when I met him at a diner in North Kansas City for my very first interview with him in 1993.*

—Paul Black, *Cerner* chief operating officer[1]

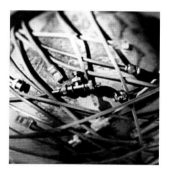

I N THE 21ST CENTURY, *CERNER* continues to develop the next generation of healthcare information technology, never wavering from its original mission of improving the safety and efficiency of healthcare delivery.

With the company's three founders at the helm, *Cerner* has established itself as the industry leader and been hailed as one of the most innovative and forward-looking technology companies in the world. *Cerner*'s commitment to revolutionizing the industry continues with an ever-increasing financial investment in research and development to create the futuristic solutions that will define the coming sea change of healthcare IT.

"Innovation is the core of what we do, and our commitment to R&D [research and development] is reflected in the fact that we've invested over a billion dollars into it since the mid-'90s and are on track to invest another billion in the next five to six years," said Allan Kells, director of investor relations. He continued:

We have consistently invested more in R&D than our peers and proven the ability to use those investments to fuel Cerner's *growth.*

With our consistent investment in technology, we have grown our revenues, have grown the company at a much greater rate than any of our peers over long periods of time. We've grown the company on average 20 percent a year for the past 10 years. That's a long-standing record of creating growth by investing in intellectual property.[2]

New global clients and climbing sales of Millennium solutions in the early 2000s prompted *Cerner* to restructure its organization in 2002. *Cerner*, which was recognized that year as the largest independent healthcare IT company in the world, had more than 1,600 clients worldwide using 1,700 active Millennium solutions.[3]

Patterson met with executives in the summer and fall of 2002 to discuss a more efficient operational structure to provide sales and support to the company's expanding number of clients.[4] The new outlay divided the company's presence around the world into six geographical areas, five of which are called a *Cerner* in *Cerner* (CinC). The six entities are the *Cerner* Global Organization, *Cerner* Great Lakes, *Cerner* Mid America, *Cerner* North Atlantic, *Cerner* Southeast, and *Cerner* West. By creating smaller companies with their own sales and support management, *Cerner* could stay close to its clients in every corner of the United States and the world.

"Each CinC has a president, a lead for consulting, and a lead for technologies," explained Jon

---

Cerner is well-positioned to develop networks for governments, the largest buyers of healthcare IT in the world.

CERNER DOCTRINE

PHYSICIAN SERVICES

ACCORDING TO NEAL PATTERSON, *Cerner* co-founder and CEO, the majority of doctors in the United States work in small physician practices comprised of 10 or fewer doctors.

"During *Cerner*'s first 25 years as a company, we created a great deal of value for the large and complex organizations in healthcare, such as hospitals and large clinics," said Patterson. "We are seeking to accelerate our impact in smaller physician practices in the future. Our vision for small physician practices in the United States is to create a highly scalable, next generation digital practice and to become a low-cost, high-value service provider to the U.S. physician practice market."[1]

Thus, *Cerner* has developed a set of solutions aimed at the individual physician. The resulting Physician Services are smaller-scale systems.

"One of the objectives is to get the physician community, independent of the hospital, to see *Cerner* as a very value-added solution," said Vice President John Dragovits, who referred to the scaled-down nature of these solutions as appropriate for a "retail" rather than a "wholesale" market. "We need to do something simple, standardized, and low price-able," he said.[2]

Of *Cerner*'s renewed focus on smaller, community establishments, *Cerner* Chief of Staff Jeff Townsend said, "Even though it's a huge part of our GDP, healthcare is basically a local phenomenon. Going forward, I think we're going to see *Cerner* develop more local relationships or special business arrangements."[3]

Doolittle, *Cerner*'s transformation consultant. "The CinCs are a geographic, client-centered alignment of the company's resources. So it forces, for example, *Cerner* Mid-America to grow its capabilities because *Cerner* Mid-America has clients with particular needs, and you have to fill them from within your CinC. Each CinC must understand the needs of its clients and grow its business."[5]

Specific groups of troubleshooters and consultants are associated with each CinC, and Dick Flanigan, president of *Cerner* North Atlantic, emphasized that sales are perhaps the highest priority of each CinC president. "It's the No. 1 thing you have to do," he said. "If you don't grow the top line, nobody really cares about anything else."[6]

The president of each CinC is responsible for a separate profit and loss statement; therefore, all of the company's domestic business is reflected in the performance of the five CinCs.

The *Cerner* Global Organization is structured separate of CinC, with three main regions of Canada; Europe, the Middle East, and Africa (EMEA); and the Asia Pacific. Townsend explained that *Cerner*'s global operations are still growing and do not yet reflect a large portion of the company's business. "Our global business hasn't broken through the 10 percent mark for the most part," he said in 2005, "so the CinCs are 90 percent-plus of our business. We have multiple business models and channels, but at the end of the day, they all get applied to the regional model as the clients are all assigned into those regions."[7]

After the CinCs became operational in January 2003, *Cerner* Senior Vice President and General Manager Mike Valentine described the importance of a "containment" strategy in their overall performance.

"You can put your arms around the business," he said. "It's not *Cerner* in total, it's actually *Cerner* modularized into a geography. So [you] can put your arms around an entire geography and say, "Here's what we need to do to be successful in this marketplace," and then you can build teams that live in those locales, and they have a sense of community. So, instead of flying to New York one week and California another week, they know that they're going to be working in this community. They get to know other people."[8]

Even though each CinC region is not "*Cerner* in total," as part of the larger company each region

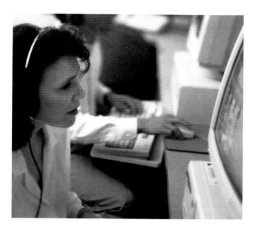 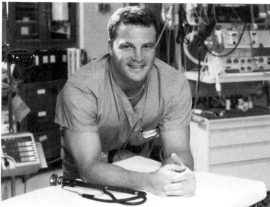 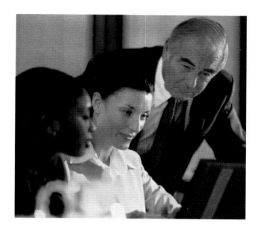

Above left: A solution in development will streamline call center operations at healthcare facilities.

Above center: Lighthouse solutions will allow hospitals to subscribe to state-of-the-art methodologies for specific medical procedures.

Above right: With its Accelerated Solutions Center, *Cerner* was the first in the industry to create a simplified, less-expensive system for implementing complex IT solutions.

has vast resources at its disposal, unlike smaller companies that have limited research and development and intellectual property.

Matt Wilson, vice president of *Cerner* Great Lakes, was struck by this difference after coming to *Cerner* from a highly creative but smaller company. There, the ideas were often good, but the structure was not in place to follow through with them. "At *Cerner*, with our culture and the discipline we've got as a leadership group, we continue fostering ideas and encouraging free thinking," he said. "At the same time, the next question is, 'That's a great idea. How do we make it work? How do we make it a reality?' It takes longer with smaller companies."[9]

Renewed Advocacy for Healthcare IT

Two events in 2004 demonstrated that healthcare IT had finally been recognized as crucial to the future of America's $1.7 trillion healthcare industry. First, President George W. Bush signed an executive order in April that created the position of the National Health Information Technology

Coordinator, a new role within the Department of Health and Human Services (HHS).

Second, the person named as coordinator of that new agency, David Brailer, was ranked by *Modern Healthcare* as No. 1 on its list of "The 100 Most Powerful People in Healthcare."[10] This distinction revealed the extent to which the industry

---

CERNER DOCTRINE

IMPLEMENTATION

TRANSFORMING A HEALTHCARE organization starts with technology delivery. This is the first strategy to launching a healthcare system towards transformation, through designing, building, testing, and delivering the plan.

Cerner's approach to event-based implementations is crucial to the transformation of healthcare. Senior Manager Jason Douthit said, "Our approach focuses on content and methodology, driving a community founded on knowledge and intellectual property. Equipped with this content, we can reduce variances in projects and ensure better outcomes for the client."[1]

The approach streamlines *Cerner*'s internal organization and clarifies project team roles, forming a fully-integrated architecture of resources.

relies on IT to solve healthcare's safety, efficiency, and financial challenges.

The goals of the office of the National Health Information Technology Coordinator echo the mission that *Cerner* has postulated throughout its 25-year history—from automating medical records to providing physicians with instant access to a knowledge database, to creating a community-wide health information infrastructure. As outlined in the executive order, the new agency was created to support the "development of a nationwide interoperable health information technology infrastructure" that does the following:

- Ensures that appropriate information to guide medical decisions is available at the time and place of care;
- Improves healthcare quality, reduces medical errors, and advances the delivery of appropriate, evidence-based medical care;
- Reduces healthcare costs resulting from inefficiency, medical errors, inappropriate care, and incomplete information;
- Promotes a more effective marketplace, greater competition, and increased choice through the wider availability of accurate information on healthcare costs, quality, and outcomes;
- Improves the coordination of care and information among hospitals, laboratories, physician offices, and other ambulatory care providers through an effective infrastructure for the secure and authorized exchange of healthcare information; and
- Ensures that patients' individually identifiable health information is secure and protected.[11]

America's new healthcare IT czar came from careers in medicine, business, and IT before being named to his new post. Brailer earned a medical degree and Ph.D. in managerial economics from the University of Pennsylvania, and served for 10 years as chairman and CEO of CareScience, a healthcare IT company based in Philadelphia. Like Patterson and other leaders in the healthcare IT industry, Brailer realizes that progress in bringing IT to healthcare has been slow, but he believes that automated systems will eventually find their place at the core of healthcare.

"I feel like I've been standing here, working on the same things for the last 15 years, and the rest of the world has finally caught up," said Brailer when he was named to the *Modern Healthcare* list. "It's no surprise that if you go back 10 years, this topic was unheard of. I used to go visit people, and they thought I was insane. Five years ago, quality of care—and information technology as a way of doing that—started to get traction. Now it's center stage."[12]

Large-scale healthcare connections as envisioned by Brailer are known at *Cerner* as state and regional "grid" systems. The regional health information organization RHIO is the broad industry label for systems that connect communities.

The Grid system is "creating a layer that sits above the four walls of either a hospital or a physician office to create the exchange of data more freely between those participants," explained Jay Linney, *Cerner*'s vice president of state and regional Grids. "There will be multiple RHIOs occurring either at a community level or a state level or regional level, and regional may be multistate, but that all ends up pulling into a national information network."[13]

One such example of a state Grid has been the venture between *Cerner* and Shared Health, a new company formed by Blue Cross Blue Shield of Tennessee, signed in May 2005. The deal proposed the use of *Cerner* solutions to connect healthcare organizations throughout Tennessee by creating a database of patients' medical records. This Community Connection database could eventually contain all health records in the state, including the government's TennCare plan. As of December 2005, more than 740,000 patients were registered under Tennessee's community health record.

Physicians, hospitals, and insurers stand to gain from the cost-cutting measures of reducing duplication, adverse drug effects, and unnecessary hospital admissions.[14] According to the *Nashville Business Journal*, savings from the creation of a centralized health record have been estimated at 20 percent.[15]

Solutions in Development

Among the projects that were on the drawing board at *Cerner* in 2005 were Millennium solutions aimed at targeting care delivery and operational management in orthopedics, pulmonology, genetics, and oncology. Another solution in the planning stages targeted facilities' call center operations, bringing more efficiency to this method of communication between the person and the healthcare provider.

Speeding up the implementation of solutions has been the focus of another program *Cerner* began developing in 2000, the Accelerated Solution Center (ASC), which was launched in response to the needs of smaller facilities that wanted a more simplified and inexpensive implementation process.

For the first two years of development, the ASC was called the Solutions Factory. "The idea was, there was a part of the market we were not addressing from an implementation or cost standpoint, and that was the community hospital market," explained Doug Abel, former vice president of the ASC. "When I took over [in 2002], we renamed it the Accelerated Solutions Center, and I began to realize that what

we were sitting on here was not just a place to address the low end of the market, but a process that was highly predictable, was focused on output, and yielded results that allowed us to go turn on more applications than we typically had done."[16]

Instead of large teams of associates going to client sites, clients come to Kansas City headquarters to participate in week-long ASC workshops. A typical client will send five teams, putting in five weeks at *Cerner*. The first week involves strong clinical participation and is attended by doctors and

Cerner's roadmap to success outlines the company's past, present, and future focus. As *Cerner* grows, the breadth of its solutions continues to expand, reaching new realms of the healthcare industry.

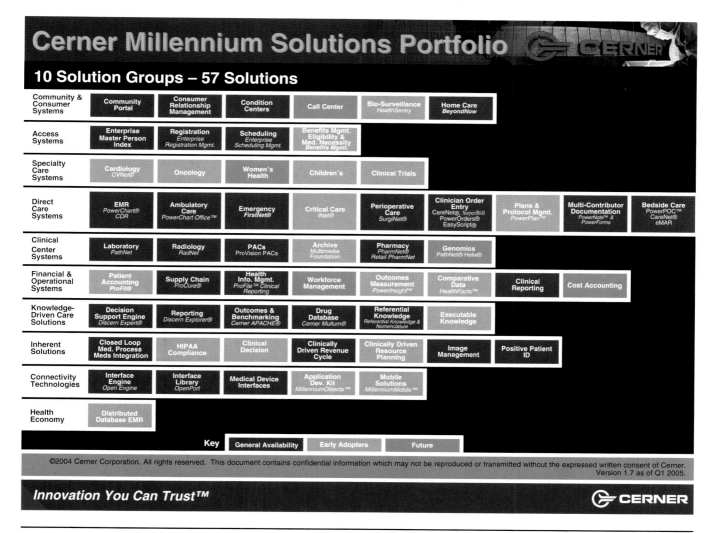

nurses who help with the design phase. The last group is made up of the hospital's IT staff, who focus on the maintenance issues of the new solutions.

Part of the streamlining in the ASC is made possible by *Cerner's* Bedrock method, which puts much of the input component of the design into the hands of *Cerner* associates. Previously, after collecting enough information to create a client-specific solution, Cerner would ask the client to enter all of the data, including rooms, beds, doctors, med-

ications, and orderables, into the system themselves. In the ASC approach, Cerner takes responsibility for that step. Thus, resources are saved since the design process is condensed. In condensing the design process, the building of applications and the implementation process, both time and resources are saved.[17]

Although the ASC was originally conceived to help keep costs down for smaller clients, *Cerner* soon discovered that the process would be valuable for

PATTERSON
RANKS AMONG POWERFUL

IN 2002, *MODERN HEALTHCARE* MAGAzine began publishing an annual list of the most influential people in healthcare. The second year, *Cerner* CEO Neal Patterson appeared near the top of this exclusive roster.

The No. 1 most powerful person on the 2003 list was President George W. Bush, and the others who preceded Patterson's No. 13 slot included Tommy Thompson, the U.S. Secretary of Health and Human Services; John Ashcroft, U.S. Attorney General; and Senators Bill Frist, Edward Kennedy, and Richard Gephart.

The list was created using input from *Modern Healthcare* readers, who were asked to nominate and vote for people they believe have the power to influence healthcare.

Patterson made the list again in 2004 and 2005.

In 2003, CEO Neal Patterson ranked 13th on *Modern Healthcare* magazine's list of the 100 most powerful people in healthcare. *(Photo courtesy of Modern Healthcare Magazine.)*

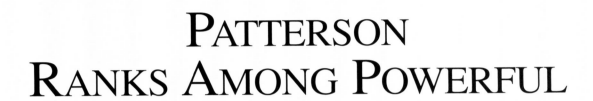

facilities of all sizes. As all clients want their infrastructure to be simpler, easier, more predictable, and less expensive, *Cerner* has extended this approach beyond the small community hospitals for use with the majority of their clients.[18]

The first client went live through an ASC implementation in 2001, and since then, about one in seven new Millennium conversions has been implemented through the ASC process. As more clients are electing to implement solutions on the ASC model instead of the field-based custom model, the traditional method of extensive on-site training and design may be reduced to a smaller fraction of clients.[19]

Although Millennium technology now comprises the mainstay of *Cerner* solutions, the company remains committed to clients who continue to use Classic. "Looking back at our Classic base, we've still got a number of engineers on the support side who are fielding questions from clients in the field and resolving issues," said Mark Schonhoff, vice president of providing care. "They are still, while not enhancing the Classic code, correcting feedback and supporting it. So we're absolutely still in a dual mode in that on the Millennium side, adding new enhancements as well as doing the support piece."[20]

Regarding the latest solutions, Schonhoff added, "There is a pretty common thought that our solutions are never done. We're continuously adding in new enhancements, as well as correcting any kinds of defects and resolving any kinds of issues in the code."[21]

Coordinated Healthcare for All

When *Cerner* began focusing on global expansion in the 1990s, it recognized that governments are the largest buyers of healthcare IT in the world. As a result, its strategy in developing systems capable of supporting national healthcare systems has been to design solutions that gather and analyze knowledge about entire populations.

According to the 1995 annual report, "*Cerner* is developing [solutions] that will aggregate vast amounts of public health information to facilitate disease management, prediction, and prevention research in support of these government purchasers. Such initiatives clearly demonstrate *Cerner*'s position as the premier information management supplier to the health industry."[22]

The first American president to advocate a universal healthcare system was Theodore Roosevelt during his two terms from 1901 to 1909. He also made national health insurance a key issue during his unsuccessful presidential election campaign of 1912. Since then, progressives in both major political parties have had little success with the issue. President Harry S. Truman included a national health insurance plan in his Fair Deal bill of 1949, which Congress did not approve, and President Richard Nixon proposed coverage for all Americans in his 1971 State of the Union Address.

In 1993, President Bill Clinton proposed a sweeping health reform package, stating to Congress that "this healthcare system is badly broken, and we need to fix it."[23] Although Clinton's plan did not even make it to a vote in Congress, it put healthcare reform squarely at the forefront of American politics.

The concept of a universal healthcare system, also known as a single-payer plan, entails coverage for everyone, similar to the Medicaid system for low-income Americans. The controversy surrounding universal coverage includes arguments against moving toward socialism and causing too great a tax burden on working people. Former U.S. Surgeon General C. Everett Koop, M.D., summed up the conflict in his comments after the Clinton plan failed in 1994:

Healthcare reform presents the greatest challenge given to a democratic republic—what's best for all of us may not be best for each of us. We say we want to be our brother's keeper, and polls show 70 percent of the citizenry is concerned about the working poor and the uninsured. But when asked if they are willing to have an income tax raise to take care of them, only 20 percent said they would.[24]

In his January 2004 State of the Union address, President George W. Bush declared his opposition to a national healthcare plan. "A government-run healthcare system is the wrong prescription," he said. "By keeping costs under control, expanding access, and helping more Americans afford coverage, we will preserve the system of private medicine that makes America's healthcare the best in the world."[25]

The universal healthcare debate is far from over, but Bush's strong support of healthcare IT as one of the solutions to making the current system more efficient has solidified the vision of industry leaders

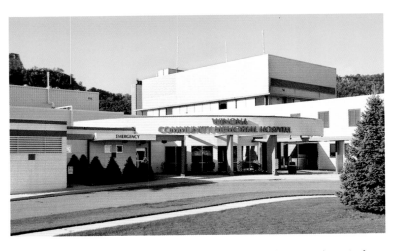

Community Memorial Hospital in Winona, Minnesota, is part of *Cerner*'s Winona Health Online project that electronically connects 30,000 residents to health information. Users can e-mail their doctors, take health-risk assessments, check for drug interactions, and access medical directories. The program will eventually include complete electronic medical records.

like Patterson. *Cerner* continues to work on expanding IT's power to connect large populations and entire communities.

In 2000, *Cerner* turned its community model into reality with the launch of Winona Health Online, a system that electronically connects every resident of Winona, Minnesota, to health information. *Cerner* teamed up with Winona Health—an organization that includes Community Memorial Hospital, pharmacies, surgical offices, and other facilities—to create an electronic personal health record (PHR).

"It was a universal vision by physicians and the hospital to have all information about our patients in the same database," said Winona Health CFO Mike Allen, "so it could be accessible wherever the patient may be, and so it could move with the patient through the health system here in Winona."[26]

Winona, with a population of approximately 30,000, was wired for the project with high-speed access provided by Hiawatha Broadband, a local company. More than 60 percent of the population has access to the Internet at home or work, and the rest of the town has access through computer labs set up at schools and senior centers.

Winona Health went through a five-step process to get the initial PHR online. First, it published the

Web site, www.winonahealthonline.org, through which the entire system would function. The site, which became active in June 2000, provides users with health tips and secure e-mail messaging to their doctors. Second, the site was updated to allow users to take health risk assessments, check for drug interactions, and access medical directories. Next, the system became a portal for doctors and other healthcare workers to transmit lab results and order prescription refills.

The system also began integrating all the information supplied by users to determine a baseline and eventually measure improvements in the health of members. Finally, in a phase that is still ongoing, the system is creating "a full consumer-based electronic medical record [that] allows healthcare professionals across the community and beyond to make treatment decisions based on complete patient information."[27]

The system, which is available to users at no charge, allows people in the community to renew prescriptions, make appointments at their doctor's office or clinic, exchange e-mail messages with their physicians, and receive lab results online through the Web site. Doctors also use the system to notify people about needed immunizations and mammograms, and to let them know about recalled medications.

Health education is an integral part of the project. Every week, for example, 24 Winona residents with diabetes enter their glucose levels and other health information into the system, and the center's educators correspond with them about the best ways to manage their disease. As of 2004, 15 of those residents had made "a significant positive health habit change, including the closer monitoring of glucose levels."[28]

In addition to connecting people to their physicians and physicians to each other, the ever-growing baseline of user information will help administrators develop new community health initiatives.[29]

Winona's groundbreaking PHR was soon followed up by additional *Cerner* solutions including *PowerChart®, PathNet®, PharmNet®, RadNet®, IQHealth™, ProVision™ PACS,* and others. Bill Davis, M.D., commented on the improvements that Winona Health Online has brought to his practice, from giving him more time with patients to streamlining his billing system.

"The biggest benefit is immediate access to the record, any place, any time," he said. "I have patients calling me at home, and I look at their record; it's right there. It's hard to beat that. And electronic prescribing is a huge advantage. All their meds are there, the interactions are documented, and it avoids errors." His practice, Family Medicine of Winona, P.A., noticed immediate results after going online with *PowerChart® Office.* "With the link into our billing, in the first year after go-live, we increased our billings by $500,000 by more accurately coding visits."[30]

One year after the launch of Winona Health Online, *Cerner* established a Scientific Advisory Board that will measure the impact of the project on the residents of Winona. The company also began working with the University of Minnesota School of Public Health and Carlson School of Management to study the project, including its impact on treating diabetes and heart disease.

In a news release announcing the new advisory board, Doug Pousma, M.D., *Cerner*'s director of *IQHealth*™, said the community system represents the future of healthcare. "This initiative represents a completely new way for consumers to improve health and prevent illness by connecting to physicians, health information, and the care delivery process.... Winona Health Online will help transform healthcare."[31]

Reports about progress made in the Winona Health Online project in 2004 coincided with several events celebrating *Cerner*'s 25th anniversary. In September, the company was honored by the Kauffman Foundation with a breakfast event at foundation headquarters. That same month, *Cerner* donated a picnic table to Kansas City's Loose Park to commemorate the three founders' first company brainstorming sessions there. The table holds a plaque that is inscribed, "To Jacob L. Loose and All of Kansas City's Great Entrepreneurs."

In October, *Cerner* participated in the annual American Royal parade in Kansas City, entering a three-section float that celebrated the company's past, present, and future. The "past" section consisted of

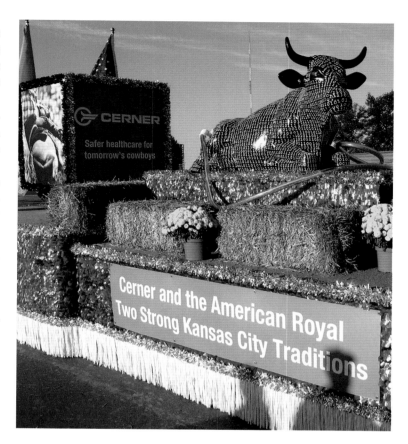

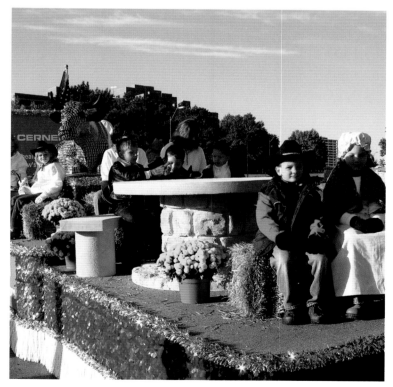

Cerner's float in Kansas City's 2004 American Royal parade featured "Digital the Cow," above, a sculpture covered with the zeroes and ones that make up binary computer code, and three young boys sitting around a picnic table, left, that represented young entrepreneurs Patterson, Gorup, and Illig.

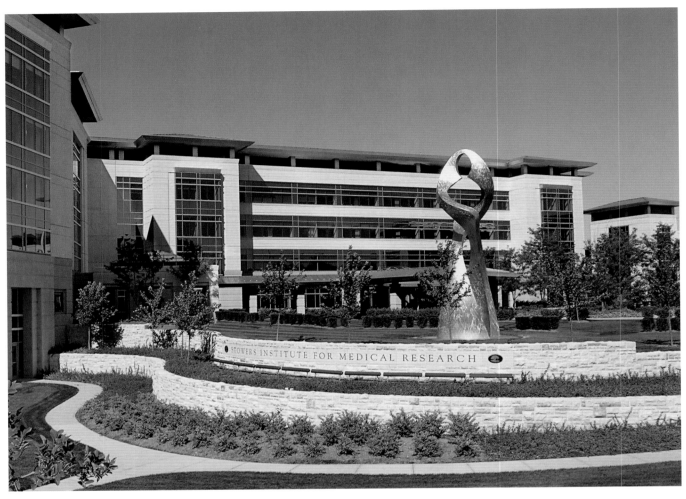

three young boys at a picnic table, representing young entrepreneur wannabees Patterson, Illig, and Gorup. In 2005, Patterson began serving as chairman of American Royal, one of the Midwest's largest events that, in addition to the parade, includes professional horse competitions, rodeos, livestock exhibitions, concerts, and the "World's Largest Barbecue Contest."[32]

Above and opposite: The Stowers Institute for Medical Research in Kansas City is dedicated to conducting research to "unlock the mysteries of disease." The Stowers Institute's 600,000-square-foot complex will eventually house up to 45 independent research programs and 500 scientists and administrative staff. (*Photos © Don Ipock.*)

Kansas City: A Hotbed of Innovation

Throughout 25 years of growth, as it forged ahead to become the leader in the global healthcare IT industry, *Cerner* brought the world's focus to its headquarters in Kansas City. Two other local organizations have also helped put the city on the map as a center of medical innovation and research.

One is the Stowers Institute for Medical Research, which "conducts basic research on genes and pro-

teins that control fundamental processes in living cells to unlock the mysteries of disease and find the keys to their causes, treatment, and prevention."[33]

The Stowers Institute was established by Jim and Virginia Stowers, founders of the Kansas City mutual funds firm American Century Companies. Virginia Stowers had worked for many years as a nurse/anesthetist, and both she and her husband are cancer survivors who chose to use their wealth to advance medical research.

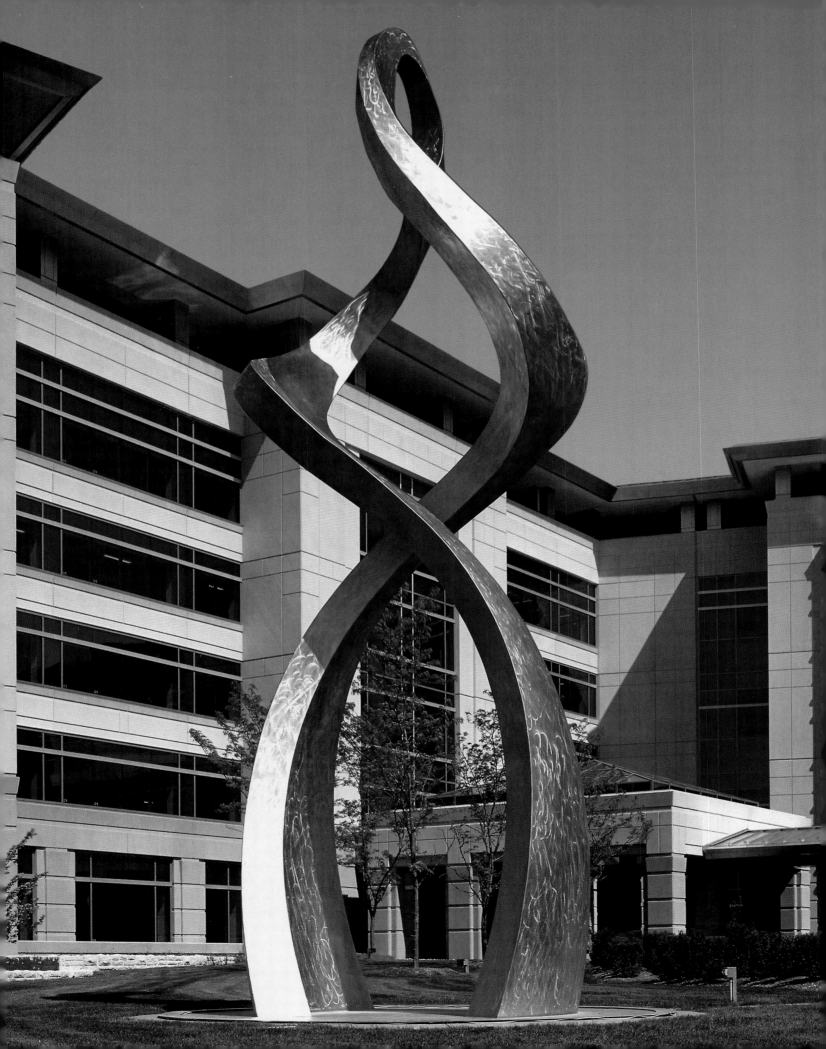

In 2000, a 600,000-square-foot, state-of-the-art complex funded by the Stowers' $1.7 billion endowment, was completed. The complex will eventually be the site of 40 to 45 independent research programs run by 500 scientists and administrative staff. The institute "aspires to be one of the most innovative biomedical research organizations in the world," and is involved in a variety of research projects. Helping to facilitate *Cerner*'s relationship with the institute is William B. Neaves, Ph.D., president of Stowers and a member of *Cerner*'s board of directors.

Among the first discoveries at the institute were new findings about the Birc6 (Bruce) gene, which inhibits cell death (apoptosis). Stowers scientist Chunying Du, Ph.D., published a study that revealed previously unknown insights into how Bruce regulates p53, a gene that suppresses tumor growth. "Bruce has long been recognized as an inhibitor of apoptosis, but until now, its method of inhibition was not clear," the journal *Medical News Today* stated in January 2005.[34]

"Dr. Du's findings answer a fundamental question of apoptosis and have implications for a wide variety of diseases," said Robb Krumlauf, Ph.D., scientific director of the Stowers Institute. "These findings are an example of the broad impact of basic research conducted at the Stowers Institute."[35]

The University of Kansas Medical Center (KUMC), which celebrated its 100th anniversary in 2005, is one of the world's leading research institutions. In keeping with its tradition of advancing the latest technologies in research, as well as education, KUMC's nursing school teamed up with *Cerner* to create a first-of-its-kind training system utilizing medical IT. The program, called Simulated E-health Delivery System (SEEDS), includes a high-tech, paperless laboratory run by Millennium solutions.

The nursing school began developing the program after the Institute of Medicine published its historic report on medical errors in 1999. School administrators sought to help their students understand the technology that would help eliminate these errors and make healthcare delivery more safe and efficient.

"For our graduating healthcare students to function completely in this electronic information age, our educational approaches must address the new skill sets and languages needed to change the way data is structured, recorded, and communicated," said Karen Miller, dean of the School of Nursing.[36]

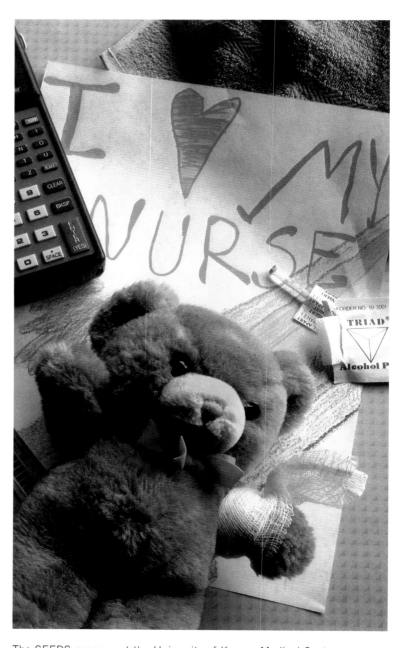

The SEEDS program at the University of Kansas Medical Center allows nursing students to gain hands-on experience with automated *Cerner* solutions.

SEEDS was ready for its first class of students in the fall of 2001. By gaining hands-on experience with various solutions in the school's simulated electronic environment, these students gained an edge when entering the workforce. "The KU School of Nursing is providing its ... graduates a competitive advantage in the marketplace," Miller said.[37]

And with the SEEDS program, *Cerner* added education to its mission of improving healthcare through IT. "Our partnership with KU's acclaimed nursing school forges a new approach to integrating clinical technology into nursing education," said *Cerner* Vice President and Chief Nursing Officer, Charlotte Weaver, R.N., Ph.D.[38]

Cerner's commitment to innovative projects such as those at the KU School of Nursing represent the innovation that has been at the heart of the company since its inception. *Cerner*'s vision for transforming healthcare was first illustrated by Patterson and Illig's cylindrical model that included layers of laboratory, clinical, and management information systems. The second image, the company's Community Health Model, envisioned how every aspect of healthcare would be electronically connected, including communications between people and their healthcare providers.

Building upon those proven models, *Cerner* conceived a maritime image for the future, which is somewhat ironic, considering the company's world headquarters is landlocked in the heart of the Midwestern United States. The model for the future includes layers of solid Bedrock, which supports a Lighthouse illuminating a vibrant prism of light.

Lighthouse is a very broad set of initiatives that encompasses two areas: harvesting and creating the content, and delivering it to clients. The content will be gathered from care providers like the Mayo Clinic, which will become the first members of the Lighthouse National Collaborative. *Cerner* summarized Lighthouse as follows:

Lighthouse is the way hospitals and clinics will optimize patient care by using data that automatically is gathered as part of the patient care flow. By creating a standard of excellence, each client can uniquely move along their quality journey, reaping the benefits of clinical process optimization. In the end, it is about achieving optimal health outcomes for our communities.[39]

Lighthouse provides clients with solutions designed for specific treatments and surgical procedures. *Cerner* has been working in partnership with major healthcare facilities, such as the Mayo

Clinic in Jacksonville, Florida, to develop Lighthouse solutions providing clients with prepackaged "methodology and content," according to *Cerner* Vice President Bryan Ince.[40]

"If you're a community hospital and you want to do a knee replacement surgery the same way they do it at Mayo," he said, "you could subscribe to that content from *Cerner*, and your Millennium system will support that methodology. You don't have to go invent it."[41]

Cerner's Bedrock initiative is part of the Lighthouse project, providing the most fundamental aspects of the design for these new solutions. Ince explained, "Bedrock puts the infrastructure of the system into place so that Lighthouse content for clinical practices can be delivered to our clients through a system, and not through countless man hours of consulting time."[42]

After *Cerner* gathers all the best-practice information about a particular procedure—such as knee replacement surgery—the design team will produce a set of options about that procedure that is tailored to each individual facility. The Bedrock element of the system will translate those options into a question-and-answer program to simplify the process of building the solution. The questions will be programmed into the Bedrock system, and the answers will automatically build the preferences and the configurations that the Millennium software looks for.[43]

The Bedrock method saves clients a great deal of time in customizing new solutions. Much of the input that has been the responsibility of clients in the past will now be performed by the design team, which will free up the user's resources. For example, the hospital's IT personnel will not need to enter such basic information as the number of doctors and nurses at the facility and the number of beds.

"The specific target is, reduce 60 percent of the effort around [the] 'design and build' [process] for our clients," said Ince, "and to be able to do a major project in three to six months."[44]

With the new layer of automation analogous here, *Cerner* symbolizes the approach to managing the healthcare continuum in a radically different way by seeking to build the infrastructure to connect the community, the region, the nation, and ultimately the globe through a series of industrial-strength grids. As the company expands its solutions

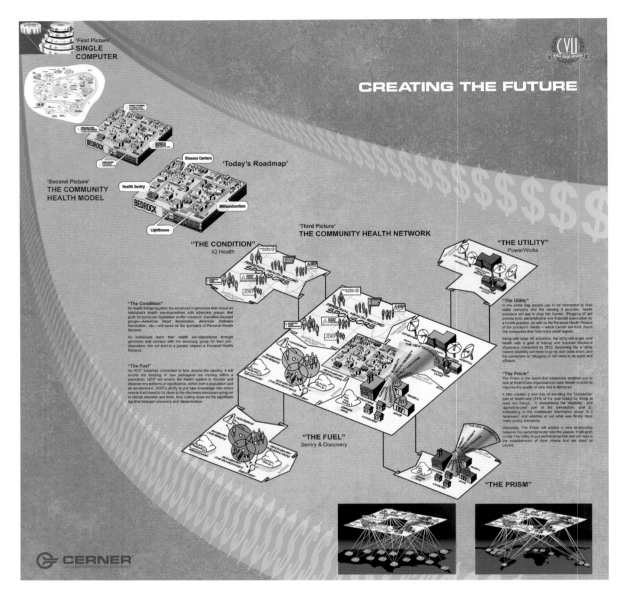

Cerner's vision for transforming healthcare was first illustrated by a cylindrical model depicting layers of laboratory, clinical, and management information systems. The second image represented the company's connected Community Health Model, and its image for the future includes layers of bedrock supporting a lighthouse. *(Image created for Cerner by 10,000 Feet, LLC.)*

into foreign countries and continues to develop systems geared toward a national scale, this global vision of transformation is becoming a reality.[45]

The two primary architects of the Lighthouse dynamic of this new model are *Cerner* founder Paul Gorup and Senior Vice President of Client Leadership Bill Dwyer. "Basically," Dwyer explained, "Lighthouse says, when hospital and health systems are fully penetrated with the electronic record in every platform—laboratory, radiology, pharmacy, notes, nursing notes, doctors notes, physician ordering—as a physician you will start thinking differently because of the explosion of information about how you will treat your patients. So Lighthouse is a concept that is patient-centric and disease/condition-specific."[46]

The model for this project has been created between *Cerner* and Jacksonville's Mayo Clinic, a major healthcare facility in the southeast, using one surgical procedure, total knee arthroplasty (TKA) as the focus to connect all the solutions. The facility is using its paperless system to build a model that identifies potential bottlenecks.

"The model, instead of going through paper and chart reviews to try to determine 'How did we treat knees this past year?', it's all automated," Dwyer said. "So you have a model that's been created by a recognized leader, and then you have the ability to map that against the practice and community hospital. Then the community hospital, if they are looking for a quality improvement, has the ability to use this model to find where those hot zones are for them. If they want to look at safety, patient safety, or if they want to look at cost, it's fully integrated and interfaces with the Millennium platform of solutions. Lighthouse is a 10-year build. I believe it will take us about that long. It's a really revolutionary idea of data management around the individual person with a disease."[47]

Future-Speak

Speculating nearly 20 years ago about life in the 21st century, science fiction writer Arthur C. Clarke wrote that the most far-reaching change in medical care would be "the complete computerization of the hospital." In Arthur C. Clarke's *July 20, 2019: Life in the 21st Century*, Clarke set the scene for the hospital of the future: "In hospital billing departments, nurses' stations, medical labs, and at patients' bedsides, the ever-present computer will process, monitor, record, and retrieve all vital information, in effect becoming the 'collective conscious' of the entire hospital."[48]

This scene began to play out in hospitals long before Clarke's remarkable scenario of the year 2019. Taking his idea to the next level, Clarke also looked beyond human-manipulated technology and pondered where robots might figure in the future of healthcare. He wrote:

It seems as if the computer's abilities are almost limitless. If so, will the computer eventually replace the practitioner? Are we swiftly approaching the day when a robot will take our temperature and blood pressure, listen to our lungs, swab our throats and do the blood workup, and then feed its data into a computer, which will in turn spit out the diagnosis?[49]

Again, Clarke's imagination was on cue, at least regarding one point-of-care experience. In 2004, five hospitals began testing robots nicknamed "robo docs" designed to roll into the hospital room to create a new type of communication between doctor and patient. At Baltimore's Johns Hopkins University, for example, surgeon Louis Kavoussi appeared in real time via a flat-screen TV attached to the robot, and viewed and listened to his patient on his computer monitor from a remote location.

Although this doctoring-from-a-distance may sound cold and technical, people were open to the idea. "So far, most patients are telling researchers that they prefer their own doctor talking to them through the robot than a stranger who happens to be in the hospital when a consultation is needed after surgery," wrote Robert Davis in *USA Today*.[50]

Other innovative trends are rapidly developing in the new millennium, such as physiologic monitoring, genotyping, and using microarrays.

In this new digital age, increasing mobility of vital information and knowledge about conditions also is being brought to the healthcare industry. Today's digital lab and radiology solutions, for example, may be developed into electronic diagnosis systems in which the computer software will make an initial diagnosis based on digital information found in the electronic medical record. The doctor could then read through the findings to confirm the diagnosis.[51]

Remote monitoring, in which sensors implanted in the human body transfer data to a computer system via a wireless connection, is another new technology that may expand into widespread use. Currently, one company has developed an implant device for people with cardiac pacemakers that transmits information about the person's heart directly to the physician. With this device, the doctor can even administer an electric shock to restart the person's heart, if needed.[52]

Information technology will also play a central role in advancing the new science of gene therapy by speeding up the process of analyzing genes. The continued sophistication of gene microarrays—many genes arranged in a regular pattern—will help scientists develop vaccines for diseases inherent in specific genes, and realize many other advances in a new era of personalized, genetically customized medicine.[53]

This is another area that *Cerner* has already addressed. "From a laboratory side, we've introduced

PathNet® Helix, which is a full genomic solution for the laboratory," said J.P. Fingado, vice president and general manager of *Cerner*'s Clinical Centers. Fingado continued:

This is an example of innovation versus being reactionary. What's happening now in the labs is the lab testing is shifting from being more of the old traditional testing—the bloods, the tissues—to actually now testing molecules and proteins. We can actually take that information and share it across all the Cerner *solutions. We'll be able to [identify] specific drug responses based on the molecular results of a person.*

You can imagine it this way: Let's say I know that I have a severe reaction to a specific drug, and my child shows up in the emergency room, and I'm not there. They're about to prescribe the drug that I have an adverse effect to. Cerner, *actually based on family-person linking, can look at the father or the mother to the child, and actually know based on molecular information what is genetically passed down and actually block that drug being given to the child. The autology will allow us to actually take genomics and spread it across all* Cerner *solutions, and, as you can imagine, this is probably the most rapidly growing area in laboratory testing over the next five years.*[54]

In the field of digital imaging, in which *Cerner* has a strong presence with solutions such as *ProVision*™ *PACS*, future advancements will include the ability of software to interpret images as well as to display them. Recent studies have established that machine-read mammograms can detect more lesions and stage them more accurately than do human radiologists.[55]

Many predict that medical IT will eventually revolutionize the way healthcare is practiced by putting more information in the hands of people, in their own homes. Just as *Cerner*'s Winona Health Online project is now proving, healthcare IT can connect entire populations to the information and professional care they need in order to take better control of their healthcare. This will allow patients and their families to have more control over their own lives and health, as well as enable them to manage their relationship with their doctors, hospitals, pharmacies, and the rest of the health system.[56]

Since its beginnings in the mid-1980s, *Cerner* has established itself as one of the most innovative IT companies in the world, with a visionary leader who was, and remains, ahead of his time. One of the traits that makes Patterson stand out is his ability to combine his software engineering knowledge with a talent for seeing the big picture.

Cerner's Paul Black, executive vice president and chief operating officer, said Patterson sees as many challenges ahead as *Cerner* has already begun to tackle. "An important part of *Cerner*'s future is to make sure that we continue to innovate. There's never a dull moment here. CEO Neal Patterson is as engaged and intense today as he was when I met him at a diner in North Kansas City for my very first interview with him in 1993."[57]

In their book, *Built to Last: Successful Habits of Visionary Companies*, James C. Collins and Jerry I. Porras defined the criteria for visionary, versus merely successful companies. "Visionary companies are premier institutions—the crown jewels—in their industries, widely admired by their peers and having a long track record of making a significant impact on the world around them."[58] The authors also described these companies as organizations that attain "extraordinary long-term performance," and have also "woven themselves into the very fabric of society."[59]

As the United States' leading healthcare IT company, *Cerner* meets these criteria and continues to set new standards for the industry. In one of the most recent examples, the Accelerated Solutions Center was launched four years before any competitors began designing similar methods for streamlining the solution implementation process.

Cerner is also a long-term performer, consistently growing in size, scope, and sales throughout its 25-year history. The company makes its mark in the fabric of society by transforming the way individuals communicate with their healthcare providers, allowing them to access and update their electronic medical records from their home computers.

Cerner also fits the profile of the authors' visionary company by focusing not on beating the competition, but on competing with itself. To the visionary company, staying ahead of the competition is not the end goal, but a byproduct of "relentlessly asking the question 'How can we improve ourselves to do better tomorrow than we did today?' No matter how much they achieve—no matter how far in front of their competitors they pull—they never think they've done 'good enough.'"[60]

In no area is this trait more evident than in *Cerner*'s enormous investment in research and development in pursuit of its mission to improve healthcare. As of 2004, *Cerner* had spent more than $1 billion in research and development, and it expects to spend an additional $1 billion through 2009.[61]

This is solid proof that the company's focus is firmly grounded in fixing healthcare's problems, and the subsequent success that the company enjoys is just one outcome of this remarkable commitment.

"When you're able to bridge information technology with medical technology, then you clearly have a chance to change the world." said *Cerner* President Trace Devanny. "My belief is that *Cerner* will be one of those companies that will be clearly recognized as a world leader in delivering the types of solutions that have made a huge impact on not only the quality of care but also the cost of care."[62]

Cerner board member Mike Herman put another number to the impact he believes *Cerner* will have on the future of healthcare. "I think one of the reasons I serve and the others do is, I really think we have the ability to change how healthcare

is being done in the United States and the world. If *Cerner* does what it thinks it can do, it could possibly lower the cost of healthcare 40 percent. Wouldn't that be wonderful?"[63]

Nancy-Ann DeParle, a member of *Cerner*'s board of directors since 2001 and former administrator of the Health Care Financing Administration (now the Centers for Medicare & Medicaid Services), is one of the country's top public policy experts and is well aware of *Cerner*'s role in transforming healthcare in the United States. She predicts that the company will remain at the forefront of the innovations necessary to move toward a safer and more efficient healthcare system.

"We're at an exciting turning point in the drive to improve the safety and quality of healthcare," DeParle said. "It's been a long journey as clinicians, hospitals, consumers, payers, and policymakers have moved from beginning to acknowledge the problems only a few years ago to today agreeing that quality of care must be measured and improved. We still have a long way to go, but we are now poised to make some great leaps forward. *Cerner* will continue to be in the vanguard of this effort—prodding all the stakeholders, developing great systems, and leading the way to a safer, better healthcare future."[64]

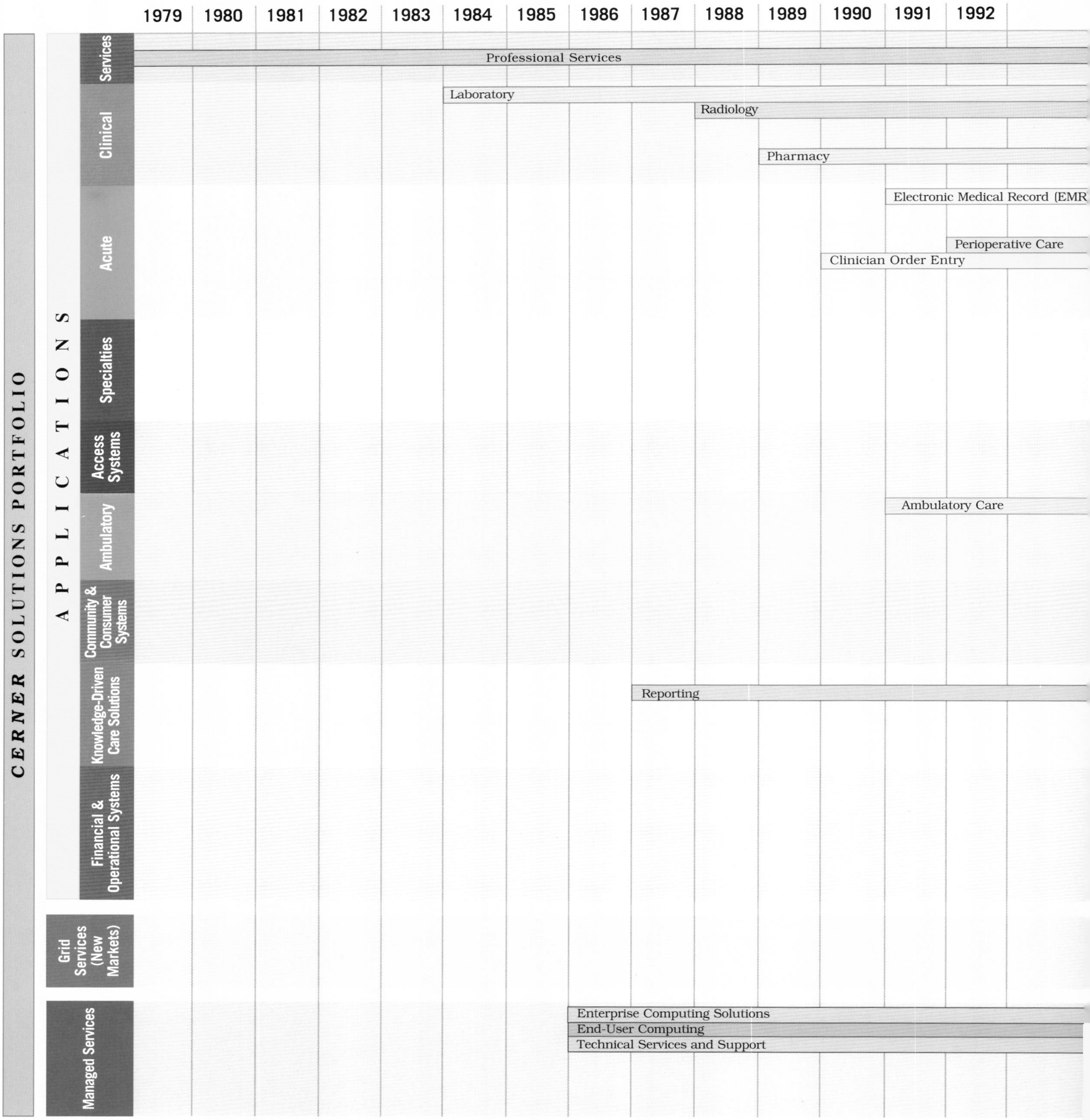

CERNER SOLUTIONS PORTFOLIO

APPLICATIONS

	1979	1980	1981	1982	1983	1984	1985	1986	1987	1988	1989	1990	1991	1992

Services

Professional Services

Clinical

Laboratory

Radiology

Pharmacy

Electronic Medical Record (EMR

Acute

Perioperative Care

Clinician Order Entry

Specialties

Access Systems

Ambulatory

Ambulatory Care

Community & Consumer Systems

Knowledge-Driven Care Solutions

Reporting

Financial & Operational Systems

Grid Services (New Markets)

Managed Services

Enterprise Computing Solutions

End-User Computing

Technical Services and Support

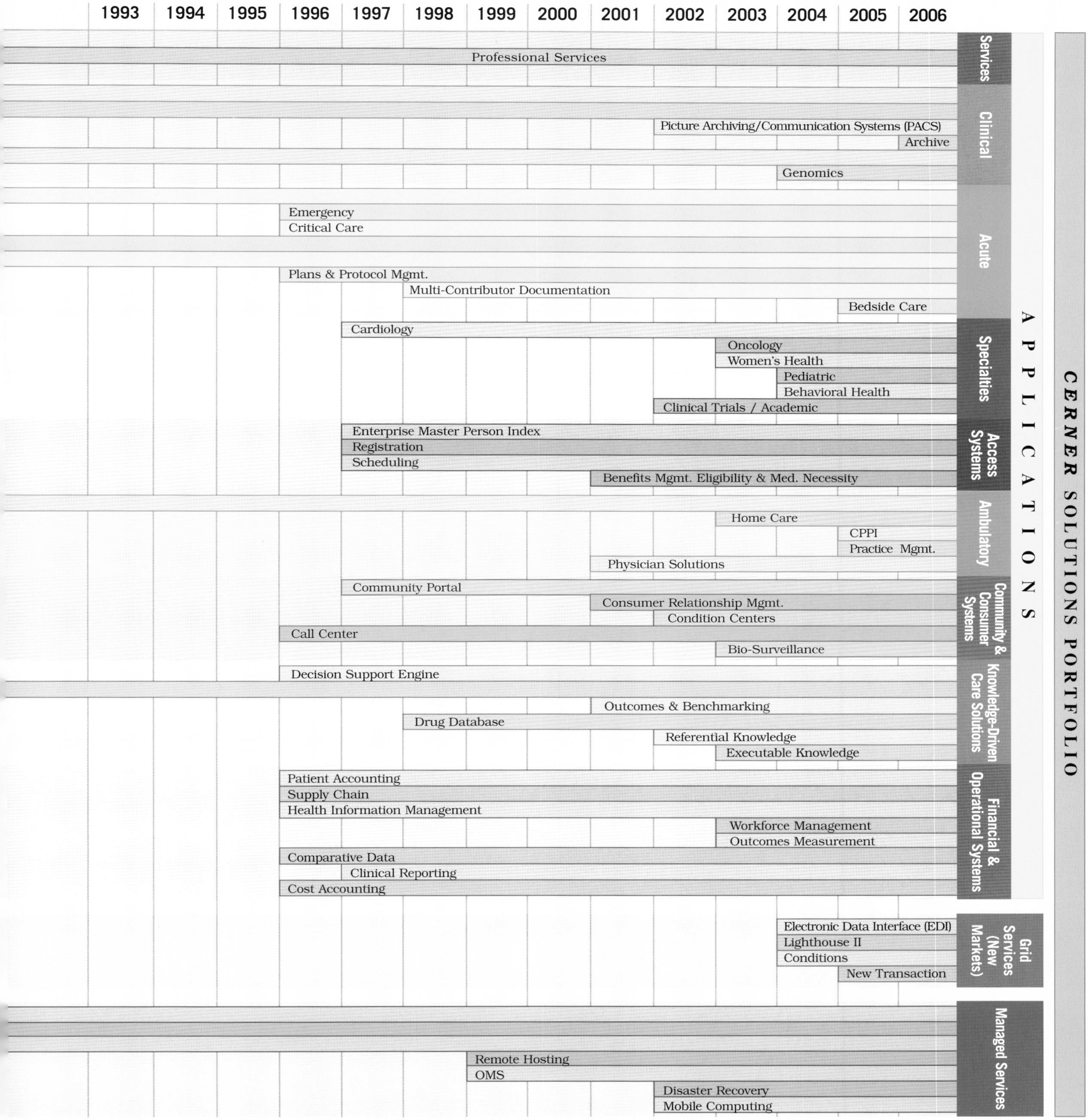

CERNER SOLUTIONS PORTFOLIO

APPLICATIONS

Years: 1993 | 1994 | 1995 | 1996 | 1997 | 1998 | 1999 | 2000 | 2001 | 2002 | 2003 | 2004 | 2005 | 2006

Services
- Professional Services

Clinical
- Picture Archiving/Communication Systems (PACS)
- Archive
- Genomics

Acute
- Emergency
- Critical Care

Specialties
- Plans & Protocol Mgmt.
- Multi-Contributor Documentation
- Bedside Care
- Cardiology
- Oncology
- Women's Health
- Pediatric
- Behavioral Health
- Clinical Trials / Academic

Access Systems
- Enterprise Master Person Index
- Registration
- Scheduling
- Benefits Mgmt. Eligibility & Med. Necessity

Ambulatory
- Home Care
- CPPI
- Practice Mgmt.
- Physician Solutions

Community & Consumer Systems
- Community Portal
- Consumer Relationship Mgmt.
- Condition Centers
- Call Center
- Bio-Surveillance

Knowledge-Driven Care Solutions
- Decision Support Engine
- Outcomes & Benchmarking
- Drug Database
- Referential Knowledge
- Executable Knowledge

Financial & Operational Systems
- Patient Accounting
- Supply Chain
- Health Information Management
- Workforce Management
- Outcomes Measurement
- Comparative Data
- Clinical Reporting
- Cost Accounting

Grid Services (New Markets)
- Electronic Data Interface (EDI)
- Lighthouse II
- Conditions
- New Transaction

Managed Services
- Remote Hosting
- OMS
- Disaster Recovery
- Mobile Computing

NOTES TO SOURCES

Chapter One

1. " 'Health Care is Broken,' *Cerner* Says," *Kansas City Star*, 23 October 2002.
2. Liane Lance, interview by Jeffrey L. Rodengen, audio recording, 1 July 2004, Write Stuff Enterprises.
3. Ibid.
4. "Neal," *Cerner Corporation 20th Anniversary Company Meeting Video*, 1999.
5. Ibid.
6. Ibid.
7. Ibid.
8. "One-time Farm Boy Heads Top Computer Corporation," *Liberty Dispatch-Tribune*, 10 April 1996.
9. "These Little Piggies Hit the Web," *Kansas City Star*, 1 November 2002.
10. Scott A. Russell, "Prominent Pikes," Pi Kappa Alpha Web site, www.pka.org/wpppat.html.
11. Rick Fiske, interview by Jeffrey L. Rodengen, audio recording, 1 July 2004, Write Stuff Enterprises.
12. *Distinguished Citizenship Award 2003, Cerner* Corporation video.
13. Ibid.
14. Ibid.
15. "Neal," *Cerner Corporation 20th Anniversary.*
16. Paul Gorup, e-mail correspondence, 22 September 2004, Write Stuff Enterprises.
17. Rick Fiske, e-mail correspondence, 31 August 2004, Write Stuff Enterprises.
18. Ibid.
19. Ibid.
20. "Neal," *Cerner Corporation 20th Anniversary.*
21. Ibid.
22. "Cliff," *Cerner Corporation 20th Anniversary Company Meeting Video, Cerner* Corporation, 1999.
23. Ibid.
24. Ibid.
25. "Neal," *Cerner Corporation 20th Anniversary.*
26. Neal Patterson, "Neal Note: Silver Top Table," *Cerner* Corporation company-wide e-mail, 8 September 2004.
27. Ibid.
28. "Neal," *Cerner Corporation 20th Anniversary.*
29. Patterson, "Neal Note: Silver Top Table."
30. "Cliff," *Cerner Corporation 20th Anniversary.*
31. "Neal," *Cerner Corporation 20th Anniversary.*
32. Ibid.
33. Ibid.
34. Lance, interview.
35. "Neal," *Cerner Corporation 20th Anniversary.*
36. Edward H. Shortliffe and Leslie E. Perreault, eds., *Medical Informatics: Computer Applications in Health Care* (New York: Addison-Wesley, 1990), 20.
37. Morris Frank Collen, M.D., *A History of Medical Informatics in the United States: 1950 to 1990* (Indianapolis: American Medical Informatics Association, 1995), 44.
38. "A Brief History of NLM," National Library of Medicine-National Institutes of Health Web site, www.nlm.nih.gov/about/briefhistory.html, 10 May 2004.
39. H. Hollerith, "An Electric Tabulating System," *The Quarterly*, Columbia University School of Mines, Vol. X No.16, (April 1889), 238-255, posted on "Columbia University Computing History" by Frank da Cruz,

www.columbia.edu/acis/
history/hh/index.html, 15
August 2004.

40. Collen, 4-5.
41. Bruce I. Blum and Karen
    Duncan, eds., *A History of
    Medical Informatics* (New York:
    ACM, 1990), 70.
42. Collen, 293-296.
43. Collen, 286, 289, 291.
44. Paul Gorup, interview by Jeffrey
    L. Rodengen, audio recording,
    10 August 2004, Write Stuff
    Enterprises.
45. Ibid.
46. Collen, 173-174.
47. Blum and Duncan, 149.
48. Collen, 184.
49. Lance, interview.
50. Linda T. Kohn, Janet M.
    Corrigna, Molla S. Donaldson,
    eds., Committee on Quality
    Health Care in America, Institute
    of Medicine, *To Err Is Human:
    Building A Safer Health System*
    (Washington, DC: National
    Academy Press, 2000), 1.
51. Robert M. Wachter, M.D., and
    Kaveh G. Shojania, M.D.,
    *Internal Bleeding: The Truth
    Behind America's Terrifying
    Epidemic of Medical Mistakes* (New
    York: Rugged Land, 2004), 56.
52. Lucian Leape, M.D., ABC News
    Good Morning America, 30
    November 1999.
53. Ibid.
54. Neal Patterson, "The Mission of
    IT in Health Care," *Healthcare
    Information Management
    Systems*, 3rd ed. (New York:
    Springer, 2004), 4.
55. Kohn, Corrigna and Donaldson, 3.
56. Liane Lance, *A Patient's
    Perspective, Cerner*
    Corporation video.
57. "'Health Care is Broken.'"
58. *Cerner* Corporation, *1986
    Annual Report.*

**Chapter One Sidebar:
An Introduction to *Cerner* Doctrines**

1. Cliff Illig, from a presentation at a
   Cerner Virtual University retreat,
   Fall 2004.
2. Paul Black, interview by Jeffrey L.
   Rodengen, audio recording, 30
   August 2005, Write Stuff
   Enterprises.

**Chapter One Sidebar:
The Most Dangerous Medical Device:
The Pen?**

1. Patterson, "The Mission of IT in
   Health Care," 17.
2. *Cerner* Corporation, *2003 Annual
   Report.*

Chapter Two

1. "On the Leading Edge, *Cerner* is
   Ready for Tomorrow," *Healthcare
   Computing & Communications*,
   June 1987.
2. "Neal," *Cerner Corporation 20th
   Anniversary.*
3. Ibid.
4. *1986 Annual Report.*
5. *Cerner* Corporation, *IPO
   Prospectus*, 5 December 1986, 16.
6. Gay Johannes, e-mail correspondence, 31 August 2004, Write
   Stuff Enterprises.
7. Lance, e-mail correspondence, 27
   September 2005, Write Stuff
   Enterprises.
8. *1986 Annual Report.*
9. Ibid.
10. "Neal," *Cerner Corporation 20th
    Anniversary.*
11. Ibid.
12. Terry Dolan, interview by Jeffrey
    L. Rodengen, audio recording,
    28 October 2004, Write Stuff
    Enterprises.
13. Ibid.

14. Ibid.
15. James Flynn, interview by
    Jeffrey L. Rodengen, audio
    recording, 5 October 2004, Write
    Stuff Enterprises.
16. Ibid.
17. Ibid.
18. Ibid.
19. Ibid.
20. Ibid.
21. Ibid.
22. Jim Mongan, interview by
    Jeffrey L. Rodengen, audio
    recording, 3 February 2005,
    Write Stuff Enterprises.
23. Ibid.
24. Janice Woods, interview by
    Jeffrey L. Rodengen, audio
    recording, 5 October 2004, Write
    Stuff Enterprises.
25. Cliff Illig, interview by Jeffrey L.
    Rodengen, audio recording, 5
    November 2004, Write Stuff
    Enterprises.
26. Woods, interview.
27. Ibid.
28. Fiske, interview.
29. Ibid.
30. Neal Patterson, interview by
    Jeffrey L. Rodengen, audio
    recording, 11 August 2004,
    Write Stuff Enterprises.
31. Ibid.
32. "Neal," *Cerner Corporation 20th
    Anniversary.*
33. Ibid.
34. Ibid.
35. Ibid.
36. Ibid.
37. Ibid.
38. Ibid.
39. *IPO Prospectus*, 13.
40. *IPO Prospectus*, 14.
41. Woods, interview.
42. Ibid.
43. Ibid.
44. Loran Walker, "Who Are Those
    Guys at *Cerner* Corporation?"
    Healthcare Computing &

Communications, August 1986, 70.
45. Ibid.
46. Ibid.
47. Ibid.
48. *Cerner* Corporation, *1988 Annual Report.*
49. Ibid.

Chapter Two Sidebar:
***Cerner* Reflects Company's Vision**

1. "Neal," *Cerner Corporation 20th Anniversary.*

Chapter Two Sidebar:
***Cerner* Doctrine Culture**

1. *1986 Annual Report.*

Chapter Two Sidebar:
World-Class Quality

1. "*Cerner* Awarded ISO 9001:2000 Certification," *Cerner* Corporation news release, 22 January 2002.
2. Shelley Looby, interview by Jeffrey L. Rodengen, 29 September 2004, Write Stuff Enterprises.

Chapter Three

1. Lance, interview.
2. *A Christmas Story, Cerner* Corporation video, 2002.
3. Ibid.
4. Ibid.
5. Ibid.
6. Bryan Ince, e-mail correspondence, 20 October 2004. Write Stuff Enterprises.
7. Anne Morgan, *Prescription for Success: The Life and Values of Ewing Marion Kauffman* (Kansas City: Andrews and McMeel, 1995), 56, 58.
8. "Kauffman Foundation: Ewing Marion Kauffman," Kauffman Foundation Web site,

www.emkf.org/pages/33.cfm, 2004.
9. "Kauffman Foundation: Who We Are," Kauffman Foundation Web site, www.kauffman.org/pages/31.cfm, 2004.
10. Neal Patterson, comments at the Kauffman Foundation's "*Cerner* in Kansas City: Celebrating a Quarter Century of Entrepreneurial Success" event, 8 September 2004.
11. Ibid.
12. Morgan, ix.
13. Ibid.
14. *Distinguished Citizenship Award 2003.*
15. Morgan, viii.
16. Ibid.
17. Mike Herman, comments at the Kauffman Foundation's "*Cerner* in Kansas City: Celebrating a Quarter Century of Entrepreneurial Success" event, 8 September 2004.
18. Carl Schramm, comments at the Kauffman Foundation's "*Cerner* in Kansas City: Celebrating a Quarter Century of Entrepreneurial Success" event, 8 September 2004.
19. Fiske, interview.
20. Herman, "*Cerner* in Kansas City."
21. Richard Tate, "Case Study: Northland School-to-Center Partnership, Kansas City, Missouri," *Innovative Local Development Programs,* www.eda.gov/PDF/1g3_1_innovldep/pdf, November 1999.
22. Morgan, x.
23. "Top Ten Reasons," *Cerner* Corporation Web site, www.cerner.com/aboutcerner/careers, 2004.
24. Patterson, "Neal Note: Silver Top Table."

25. Lance, interview.
26. Gail Blanchard, interview by Jeffrey L. Rodengen, audio recording, 2 July 2004, Write Stuff Enterprises.
27. Ibid.
28. Ibid.
29. Debbie Yantis, interview by Jeffrey L. Rodengen, audio recording, 5 January 2005, Write Stuff Enterprises.
30. Seth Rupp, interview by Jill Gambill, audio recording, 16 September 2005, Write Stuff Enterprises.
31. Mike Neal, interview by Jeffrey L. Rodengen, audio recording, 10 December 2004, Write Stuff Enterprises.
32. Francie McNair-Stoner, interview by Jeffrey L. Rodengen, audio recording, 3 December 2004, Write Stuff Enterprises.
33. Betsy Solberg, interview by Jeffrey L. Rodengen, audio recording, 15 February 2005, Write Stuff Enterprises.
34. Alan Deitrich, interview by Jeffrey L. Rodengen, audio recording, 31 January 2005, Write Stuff Enterprises.
35. Julie Wilson, interview by Jeffrey L. Rodengen, audio recording, 18 March 2005, Write Stuff Enterprises.
36. Mike Nill, interview by Jeffrey L. Rodengen, audio recording, 14 December 2004, Write Stuff Enterprises.
37. Patterson, "*Cerner* in Kansas City."
38. Ibid.
39. Blanchard, interview.
40. Ibid.
41. Ibid.
42. Ibid.
43. Owen Straub, interview by Jeffrey L. Rodengen, audio recording, 2 July 2004, Write Stuff Enterprises.

44. Dick Flanigan, interview by Jeffrey L. Rodengen, audio recording, 2 July 2004, Write Stuff Enterprises.
45. Ibid.
46. Ibid.
47. Kim Stevens, interview by Jeffrey L. Rodengen, audio recording, 14 September 2004, Write Stuff Enterprises.
48. Ibid.
49. Ibid.
50. Ibid.
51. Mark Brewer, e-mail correspondence, 10 August 2004, Write Stuff Enterprises.
52. Robert Campbell, interview by Jeffrey L. Rodengen, audio recording, 2 July 2004, Write Stuff Enterprises.
53. *Cerner* Corporation, "Traditions" presentation materials.
54. Ibid.
55. Campbell, interview.
56. Ibid.
57. Ibid.
58. *Cerner* Corporation, *1996 Annual Report.*
59. Ibid.
60. *Cerner* Corporation, *1997 Annual Report.*
61. Paul Sinclair, interview by Jeffrey L. Rodengen, audio recording, 8 December 2004, Write Stuff Enterprises.
62. Fiske, interview.
63. *Cerner* Corporation, *1992 Annual Report.*
64. Ibid.

Chapter Three Sidebar: The D³ Blooper

1. Straub, interview.

Chapter Four

1. "*Cerner* Chooses Rockcreek," *Kansas City Star*, 21 January 1994, B8.

2. *Cerner* Corporation, *Cerner Health Conference Daily News*, 11 September 2001, 1.
3. "*Cerner*'s Vital Signs," *Kansas City Star*, 7 September 1999, D11.
4. Gay Johannes, interview by Jeffrey L. Rodengen, audio recording, 1 July 2004, Write Stuff Enterprises.
5. Steve Oden, interview by Jeffrey L. Rodengen, audio recording, 2 July 2004, Write Stuff Enterprises.
6. Todd Downey, interview by Jeffrey L. Rodengen, audio recording, 2 July 2004, Write Stuff Enterprises.
7. Ibid.
8. *IPO Prospectus*, 21.
9. "*Cerner* Chooses Rockcreek."
10. Ibid.
11. Ibid.
12. Ibid.
13. Ibid.
14. "*Cerner* Corp. Expanding to Lee's Summit," *The Business Journal* (Kansas City), 25 February 2000.
15. Ibid.
16. "*Cerner* Training Center Opens in Former Casino," *Kansas City Star*, 20 April 2002.
17. "Dedicated to the Future," *Kansas City Star*, 8 October 2003, C1.
18. Ibid.
19. Ibid.
20. "*Cerner* Corp. Files for Public Stock Offering," *Kansas City Star*, 25 October 1986.
21. "Cliff," *Cerner Corporation 20th Anniversary.*
22. Ibid.
23. Ibid.
24. *IPO Prospectus*, 5.
25. Ibid.
26. Ibid.
27. "Cliff," *Cerner Corporation 20th Anniversary.*

28. Ibid.
29. "Companies Discover That Healthy Employees are Happier, More Productive," Corporate Fitness Works Web site, www.corporatefitnessworks.com /news/testimonials.htm.
30. Ibid.
31. "*Cerner*'s Perks Earn *Fortune*'s Praise," *Kansas City Star*, 1 January 1999, C1.
32. "*Cerner*'s Family–Friendly Work Program," WDAF News-Kansas City, 18 May 1999.
33. Ibid.
34. "100 Best Companies to Work for in America," *Fortune*, 11 January 1999.
35. "Cliff," *Cerner Corporation 20th Anniversary.*
36. Ibid.
37. Lupe Coursey, interview by Jeffrey L. Rodengen, audio recording, 2 November 2004, Write Stuff Enterprises.
38. Ibid.
39. *Cerner* Corporation, *1995 Annual Report.*
40. Campbell, interview.
41. Ibid.
42. Ibid.
43. Ibid.
44. Matt Hodes, interview by Jeffrey L. Rodengen, audio recording, 1 July 2004, Write Stuff Enterprises.
45. Ibid.
46. Campbell, interview.
47. Ibid.
48. Ibid.
49. *Cerner* Corporation, internal company announcement.
50. Rich Miller, interview by Amy Blakely, audio recording, 10 December 2004, Write Stuff Enterprises.
51. Rich Miller, interview by Jill Gambill, audio recording, 15 September 2005, Write Stuff Enterprises.

52. *Cerner* Corporation, *1993 Annual Report.*
53. Ibid.
54. John Landis, interview by Jeffrey L. Rodengen, audio recording, 29 November 2004, Write Stuff Enterprises.
55. Jack Newman Jr., interview by Jeffrey L. Rodengen, audio recording, 7 December 2004, Write Stuff Enterprises.
56. "*Cerner* Corporation," *CEO Interviews*, 29 February 1988, 2,261.
57. Ibid.
58. *1986 Annual Report.*
59. *Cerner* Corporation, *1987 Annual Report.*
60. *Cerner* Corporation, *1990 Annual Report.*
61. Ibid.
62. *Cerner* Corporation, *1998 Annual Report.*
63. Ibid.
64. "*Cerner* Predicting Pent–up Demand," *The Business Journal* (Kansas City), 23 April 1999.
65. "Synetic and *Cerner* Announce Strategic Alliance," Business Wire, 21 January 1999.
66. Jeff Townsend, interview by Jeffrey L. Rodengen, audio recording, 23 August 2005, Write Stuff Enterprises.
67. Black, interview, 30 August 2005.
68. "*Cerner* Announces Agreement to Acquire Clinical Information Systems," *Cerner* Corporation news release, www.cerner.com/public/NewsReleases_1a.asp?id=257, 15 May 2000.
69. "*Cerner* Acquires ADAC Healthcare Information Systems," *Cerner* Corporation news release, www.cerner.com/public/NewsReleases_1a.asp?id=257&cid=119, 21 November 2000.

70. "*Cerner* Completes Previously Announced Acquisition of Dynamic Healthcare Technologies, Inc.," *Cerner* Corporation news release, www.cerner.com/public/NewsReleases_1a.asp?id=257&cid=158, 17 December 2001.
71. "*Cerner* to Acquire VitalWorks' Medical Division, a Leader in Physician Office Technologies," *Cerner* Corporation news release, www.cerner.com/public/NewsReleases_1a.asp?id=257&cid=626, 16 November 2004.
72. "*Cerner* Acquires French Information Technology Company," *Cerner* Corporation news release, www.cerner.com/public/NewsReleases_1a.asp?id=257, 3 May 2005.
73. *Cerner* Corporation, *2000 Annual Report.*

**Chapter Four Sidebar:
Cerner Doctrine Vision Center**

1. Donald Trigg, interview by Jeffrey L. Rodengen, audio recording, 22 November 2004, Write Stuff Enterprises.
2. Andy Heeren, "*Cerner*'s Approach to the Vision Center," *Cerner* Corporation document, 2005.
3. Ibid.

**Chapter Four Sidebar:
Cerner Doctrine Architecture**

1. *1992 Annual Report.*

**Chapter Four Sidebar:
First Hand Foundation**

1. "Helping Hand," *Kansas City Star*, 9 October 2002.
2. "First Hand at Work," First Hand Foundation Web site,

www.firsthandfoundation.org/work.asp.
3. "No Luck at the Polls? What's a Millionaire to Do?" Associated Press, 12 November 2004.

Chapter Five

1. "*Cerner* Acquires Zynx Health, Incorporated," *Cerner* Corporation news release, www.cerner.com/aboutcerner/pressreleases.asp?id=955, 2 May 2002.
2. Illig, interview.
3. Ibid.
4. Ibid.
5. *Cerner* Corporation, *1989 Annual Report.*
6. Alexis and Richard Rognehaugh, *Healthcare IT Terms* (Chicago: Healthcare Information and Management Systems Society, 2001), 115.
7. "A Proven PACS Solution," *Cerner* Corporation Web site, www.cerner.com/products/products_4a.asp?id=1046, 2004.
8. *1989 Annual Report.*
9. Illig, interview.
10. Ibid.
11. "On the Leading Edge, *Cerner* is Ready for Tomorrow," *Healthcare Computing & Communication*, June 1987, 21.
12. Illig, interview.
13. *1990 Annual Report.*
14. *Cerner* Corporation, *1991 Annual Report.*
15. Kathleen M. Young, *Informatics for Healthcare Professionals* (Philadelphia: F.A. Davis, 2000), 97.
16. Ibid.
17. Ibid.
18. George W. Bush, "State of the Union," 20 January 2004, www.whitehouse.gov/news/releases/2004/01/20040120-7.html.

19. "Bush Touts Plan for Electronic Medicine," *The Washington Post*, 28 May 2004, A8.

20. David McCallie, interview by Jeffrey L. Rodengen, audio recording, 11 August 2004, Write Stuff Enterprises.

21. Ibid.

22. Ibid.

23. Rognehaugh, 38.

24. "University of Illinois Medical Center," *Cerner* Corporation Web site, www.cerner.com/industry/industry _4a.asp?id=1270, 2004.

25. "CPOE Reduces Error, Improves Safety at Prominent Pediatric Hospital," *Cerner* Corporation news release, www.cerner.com/public/NewsReleases_1a.asp?id=257&cid=4669, 5 December 2005.

26. Ibid.

27. "Seattle Children's Mission Makes CPOE a Priority," *Cerner* Corporation document, www.cerner.com/public/filedownload.asp?LibraryID=17960, 2004.

28. *2003 Annual Report*.

29. "*Cerner* Recognized as CPOE Leader," *Cerner* Corporation news release, www.cerner.com/aboutcerner/pressreleases.asp?id=2400, 16 October 2003.

30. "What Analysts Are Saying About Us," *Cerner* Corporation Web site, www.cerner.com/public/MillenniumSolution.asp?id=3502.

31. "The Complete IT Answer for the Acute Care Team," *Cerner* Corporation Web site, www.cerner.com/carenet, 2004.

32. Charlotte Weaver, interview by Jeffrey L. Rodengen, audio recording, 2 December 2004, Write Stuff Enterprises.

33. "Transforming the Surgery Supply Chain," *Cerner* Corporation Web site, www.cerner.com/products/products_4a.asp?id=213, 2004.

34. "Your Most Important Perioperative Instrument," *Cerner* Corporation Web site, www.cerner.com/surginet, 2003.

35. "National Hospital Ambulatory Medical Care Survey: 2002 Emergency Department Summary," Advance Data, Centers for Disease Control and Prevention, National Center for Health Statistics Web site, www.cdc.gov/nchs/data/ad/ad340.pdf, 18 March 2004.

36. "Blue Ox Medical Solutions," *Cerner* Corporation Web site, www.cerner.com/products/products _4a.asp?id=2405, 2004.

37. Ibid.

38. "DXplain," Massachusetts General Hospital Laboratory of Computer Science Web site, www.lcs.mgh.harvard.edu/dxplain.htm.

39. *1990 Annual Report*.

40. *1991 Annual Report*.

41. "Expert Systems," American Association for Artificial Intelligence Web site, www.aaai.org/AITopics.html/expert.html, 2004.

42. "Knowledge-Driven Care: An Educational White Paper," *Cerner* Corporation Web site, www.cerner.com/products/products_3a.asp?id=2676.

43. Ibid.

44. "Fact Sheet: Improving Health Care Quality," Agency for Healthcare Research and Quality Publication No. 02-P032, September 2002.

45. Ibid.

46. "Knowledge-Driven Care."

47. "*Cerner* Acquires Zynx Health, Incorporated."

48. Ibid.

49. "Knowledge Infrastructure," *Cerner* Corporation Web site, www.cerner.com/products/products_4a.asp?id=2680.

50. "Sun Health Corporation," *Cerner* Corporation Web site, www.cerner.com/products/products_4a.asp?id=2686.

51. Ibid.

52. "Executable Knowledge," *Cerner* Corporation Web site, www.cerner.com/products/products_4a.asp?id=2686.

53. *Cerner* Corporation, *2001 Annual Report*.

54. "Sarasota Memorial Hospital," *Cerner* Corporation document, www.cerner.com/products/products_4a.asp?id=2694.

55. Ibid.

56. "Health Facts," *Cerner* Corporation Web site, www.cerner.com/products/products_4a.asp?id=2692.

57. Gorup, interview.

58. Ibid.

59. "Peer Q & A: Dr. Michael Salesin," *Cerner* Corporation Web site, www.cerner.com/physicians/physicians_3a.asp?id=861.

60. "Cardiology: Testimonials," *Cerner* Corporation Web site, www.cerner.com/products/products_4a.asp?id=1043.

61. Ibid.

62. Patterson, "The Mission of IT in Health Care," 16.

63. Ibid, 17.

64. Ibid.

65. "*Cerner* Launches $25 Million, 10-Year Initiative to Provide Personal Health Records to Kids With Diabetes," *Cerner* Corporation news release, www.cerner.com/public/NewsReleases_1a.asp?id=257&cid=228, 12 October 2004.

66. "BeyondNow FAQ," *Cerner* Corporation Web site, www.cerner.com/aboutcerner/ newsroom_4a.asp?id=2261.
67. "Computer System Would Warn of Early Signs of Bioterrorist Attacks," *Kansas City Star*, 23 April 2002.
68. Ibid.
69. Oden, interview.
70. Ibid.
71. Ibid.
72. "Healthcare Intelligence," *Cerner* Corporation Web site, www.cerner.com/products/ products_4a.asp?id=359.
73. Shellee Spring, interview by Jeffrey L. Rodengen, audio recording, 1 July 2004, Write Stuff Enterprises.
74. "*Cerner* Corporation to Premiere Enterprise-Wide Clinical Image Management System at RSNA," *Cerner* Corporation news release, www.cerner.com/ aboutcerner/pressreleases. asp?id=1037, 13 November 2001.
75. Ibid.
76. Oden, interview.
77. Chris Murrish, interview by Jeffrey L. Rodengen, audio recording, 10 August 2004, Write Stuff Enterprises.

Chapter Five Sidebar:
***Cerner* Doctrine Leadership**

1. *1996 Annual Report.*

Chapter Five Sidebar:
A Person-Centered Philosophy

1. Patterson, interview.

Chapter Six

1. Mike Wright and David Rhodes, *Manage IT* (Westport: Greenwood, 1986), 86–88.

2. Patterson, "Neal Note: Silver Top Table."
3. Ibid.
4. Ibid.
5. Bryan Ince, interview by Jeffrey L. Rodengen, audio recording, 11 August 2004, Write Stuff Enterprises.
6. Ibid.
7. *1997 Annual Report.*
8. McCallie, interview.
9. Ibid.
10. Straub, interview.
11. *1997 Annual Report.*
12. *1996 Annual Report.*
13. Wright and Rhodes, 86-88.
14. Brian Streich, interview by Jeffrey L. Rodengen, audio recording, 10 August 2004, Write Stuff Enterprises.
15. Julius Karash, "*Cerner* Prepares for Growth by Using 'Marathon' Strategy," *Kansas City Star*, 8 December 1996.
16. Townsend, interview by Jeffrey L. Rodengen, audio recording, 1 July 2004, Write Stuff Enterprises.
17. Ibid.
18. Dick Brown, interview by Jeffrey L. Rodengen, audio recording, 31 January 2005, Write Stuff Enterprises.
19. Ibid.
20. Tim Zoph, interview by Jeffrey L. Rodengen, audio recording, 23 March 2005, Write Stuff Enterprises.
21. Rognehaugh, 29.
22. "HNA Millennium: The Architecture for the Next Millennium," *Cerner* Corporation brochure.
23. John Travis, interview by Jeffrey L. Rodengen, audio recording, 10 August 2004, Write Stuff Enterprises.
24. Ibid.
25. Ibid.

26. "HNA Millennium."
27. Jake Sorg, interview by Jeffrey L. Rodengen, audio recording, 11 August 2004. Write Stuff Enterprises.
28. Trace Devanny, interview by Jeffrey L. Rodengen, audio recording, 10 August 2004, Write Stuff Enterprises.
29. Ibid.
30. Townsend, interview, 1 July 2004.
31. Ibid.
32. Ibid.
33. Ibid.
34. Ibid.
35. Ibid.
36. Ibid.
37. Ince, interview, 11 August 2004.
38. *1998 Annual Report.*
39. "Brighter Outlook for *Cerner* Corp. Stock," *Kansas City Star*, 25 March 1999, C2.
40. *1998 Annual Report.*
41. "Brighter Outlook for *Cerner* Corp. Stock."
42. "*Cerner* Corporation Announces First Quarter 1999 Results," *Cerner* Corporation news release, www.cerner.com/ aboutcerner/pressreleases.asp? id=899, 21 April 1999.
43. *1997 Annual Report.*
44. Townsend, interview, 1 July 2004.
45. "Bennett Report Says Health Care, International Community at High Risk for Y2K Failures," Special Committee on the Year 2000 Technology Problem news release, www.senate.gov/~y2k/news/ pr990302.htm, 2 March 1999.
46. Carol Hull, interview by Jeffrey L. Rodengen, audio recording, 2 November 2004, Write Stuff Enterprises.
47. *Cerner* Corporation, *Cerner Y2K Readiness Guide.*
48. *Cerner* Corporation, *1999 Annual Report.*

49. "*Cerner* Corporation CEO Outlines Road to Future Success," *The Wall Street Transcript*, www.twst.com/notes/articles/jah243.html, 23 February 2000.
50. *1995 Annual Report.*
51. "*Cerner* 2000 Program Gets Director," *Kansas City Star*, 28 January 1996, F2.
52. "Area Stocks to Take a Few Lumps," *Kansas City Star*, 25 June 1996, F2.
53. "*Cerner* 2000 Program Gets Director."
54. Gorup, interview.
55. Ibid.
56. Ibid.
57. Stan Sword, interview by Jeffrey L. Rodengen, audio recording, 11 August 2004, Write Stuff Enterprises.
58. Ibid.
59. Townsend, interview, 1 July 2004.
60. Sword, interview.
61. Ibid.
62. Townsend, interview, 1 July 2004.
63. Neal Patterson, "Neal Note: *Cerner*'s 9/11 Response," *Cerner* Corporation company-wide e-mail, 17 September 2001.
64. Sword, interview.
65. *2001 Annual Report.*
66. Ibid.
67. *Cerner* Corporation, *2002 Annual Report.*
68. Ibid.
69. "*Cerner* Lowers Revenue and Earnings Guidance for First Quarter of 2003," *Cerner* Corporation news release, www.cerner.com/public/NewsReleases_1a.asp?id=257&cid=232, 3 April 2003.
70. "*Cerner* Misses Numbers, Stock Tumbles," *Health Data Management* Web site, www.healthdatamanagement.com/html/PortalStory.cfm?type=vend&DID=9983, 3 April 2003.
71. "Shareholder Suits Hit Center," *Health Data Management* Web site, www.healthdatamanagement.com/html/PortalStory.cfm?type=vend&DID=9999, 8 April 2003.
72. *2003 Annual Report.*
73. Ibid.
74. "*Cerner* Delivers Strong New Business Bookings," *Cerner* Corporation news release, www.cerner.com/aboutcerner/pressreleases.asp?id=2763.
75. *Cerner* Corporation, *4Q04 Investor Relations Report*, 4 February 2005.
76. Ibid.
77. Ibid.
78. Ibid.
79. Ibid.
80. Ibid.
81. Jefferies & Company, *Cerner* Corporation analysis, 22 March 2005.

Chapter Six Sidebar:
Balanced Budget Act Rocks Healthcare

1. "The Impact of the 1997 Balanced Budget Act on Medicare," Minnesota Medicine Web site, www.mnmed.org/publications/MnMed2000/December/Silversmith.html, December 2000.
2. "Neal," *Cerner Corporation 20th Anniversary.*

Chapter Six Sidebar:
25 Years of Innovation

1. "*Cerner* Celebrates 25 Years of Innovation," *Cerner* Corporation document.
2. Ibid.
3. Ibid.
4. Ibid.

Chapter Six Sidebar:
A New Logo for a New Era

1. "*Cerner* Logo Gets a New Look," *Cerner* Corporation memorandum, 2001.
2. "Cliff," *Cerner Corporation 20th Anniversary.*

Chapter Six Sidebar:
***Cerner* Honors and Awards**

1. "Awards," *Cerner* Corporation Web site, www.cerner.com/aboutcerner/careers_4a.asp?id=771.

Chapter Seven

1. Devanny, interview.
2. *1991 Annual Report.*
3. *1993 Annual Report.*
4. *1991 Annual Report.*
5. "Singapore Home," *Cerner* Corporation Web site, www.cerner.com/ap/default.asp?id=1827, 2004.
6. *1991 Annual Report.*
7. *1993 Annual Report.*
8. "Information Technology Systems: A Case Study," *Business Briefing: Hospital Engineering & Facilities Management*, 2004, 75.
9. David Sides, interview by Jill Gambill, audio recording, 12 September 2005, Write Stuff Enterprises.
10. Jon Doolittle, interview by Jeffrey L. Rodengen, 10 August 2004, Write Stuff Enterprises.
11. *2003 Annual Report.*
12. "Ebookings Proof of Solution Fact Sheet," *Cerner* Corporation document.
13. *2003 Annual Report.*
14. Townsend, e-mail correspondence, 4 April 2005.
15. Ibid.

16. Doolittle, interview.
17. Townsend, e-mail correspon-dence.
18. John Kuckelman, interview by Jeffrey L. Rodengen, audio recording, 5 November 2004, Write Stuff Enterprises.
19. Ibid.
20. Marc Naughton, interview by Jeffrey L. Rodengen, audio recording, 10 August 2004, Write Stuff Enterprises.
21. Sides, interview.
22. Justin Scott, interview by Jeffrey L. Rodengen, audio recording, 23 August 2005, Write Stuff Enterprises.
23. Townsend, interview, 23 August 2005.
24. "*Cerner* Acquires Image Devices, GMBH," *Cerner* Corporation news release, 20 August 2002.
25. "*Cerner* CEO Answers Attacks in Kansas City, Mo." *Kansas City Star*, 28 October 2004, C1.
26. Patterson, "Neal Note," *Cerner* Corporation company-wide e-mail, 2004.
27. "*Cerner* CEO Answers Attacks in Kansas City, Mo."
28. *1992 Annual Report.*
29. Doug Krebs, interview by Jeffrey L. Rodengen, audio recording, 7 December 2004, Write Stuff Enterprises.
30. Devanny, interview.
31. Mike Breedlove, interview by Jeffrey L. Rodengen, audio recording, 16 September 2005, Write Stuff Enterprises.
32. Ibid.

**Chapter Seven Sidebar:
Simplifying German Healthcare**

1. "Klinikum Chemnitz," *Cerner* Corporation document.

Chapter Eight

1. Paul Black, interview by Jeffrey L. Rodengen, audio recording, 3 December 2004, Write Stuff Enterprises.
2. Allan Kells, interview by Jeffrey L. Rodengen, audio recording, 5 November 2004, Write Stuff Enterprises.
3. *2002 Annual Report.*
4. Flanigan, interview.
5. Doolittle, interview.
6. Flanigan, interview.
7. Townsend, interview, 4 April 2005.
8. Mike Valentine, interview by Jeffrey L. Rodengen, audio recording, 11 August 2004, Write Stuff Enterprises.
9. Matt Wilson, interview by Jeffrey L. Rodengen, audio recording, 6 December 2004, Write Stuff Enterprises.
10. "Information=Power," *Modern Healthcare*, 23 August 2004, 6.
11. "Executive Order 13335— Incentives for the Use of Health Information Technology and Establishing the National Health Information Technology Coordinator," Federal Register, www.archives.gov/federal_register/executive_orders/2004.html, 30 April 2004.
12. "Information=Power."
13. Jay Linney, interview by Jeffrey L. Rodengen, audio recording, 14 March 2005, Write Stuff Enterprises.
14. "*Cerner*, BlueCross BlueShield of Tennessee Launch Statewide Community Health Record," *Cerner* Corporation news release, www.cerner.com/NewsReleases_1a?id=257&cid=4189, 27 May 2005.

15. "BlueCross, *Cerner* Team on Database," *Nashville Business Journal*, 20 May 2005.
16. Doug Abel, interview by Jeffrey L. Rodengen, audio recording, 23 November 2004, Write Stuff Enterprises.
17. Bryan Ince, interview by Antonia Felix, audio recording, 25 January 2005, Write Stuff Enterprises.
18. Chris Giglio, interview by Antonia Felix, audio recording, 25 January 2005, Write Stuff Enterprises.
19. Ibid.
20. Mark Schonhoff, interview by Jeffrey L. Rodengen, audio recording, 1 July 2004, Write Stuff Enterprises.
21. Ibid.
22. *1995 Annual Report.*
23. "The Health Care Debate: What Went Wrong?" *The New York Times*, 29 August 1994, A1.
24. "Q & A: C. Everett Koop," *The Atlanta Journal-Constitution*, 24 November 1994, G32.
25. Bush, "State of the Union."
26. "*Cerner* Case Study: Winona Health: Connecting the Community Improves Quality of Care," *Cerner* Corporation document, 2004.
27. "Health @ Home: Connecting the Community in Winona," *Health Management Technology*, July 2002, 26.
28. "*Cerner* Case Study: Winona Health."
29. "Minn. Town to Get Health Data Online," *Modern Healthcare*, 12 June 2000, 18.
30. "*Cerner* Case Study: Winona Health."
31. "*Cerner* IQ Health Announces Study Measuring Impact of e-Health Initiative, Winona Health Online," *Cerner* Corporation

news release, www.cerner.com/aboutcerner/pressreleases.asp?id=943, 26 February 2001.

32. "American Royal Announces 2005 Barbecue Committee Chairs," American Royal news release, www.americanroyal.com/Default.aspx?tabid=57&view=show&pressid=115, 4 February 2005.

33. "Basic Facts About the Stowers Institute," Stowers Institute Web site, www.stowers-institute.org.

34. "Stowers Researcher Answers Fundamental Question of Cell Death," *Medical News Today*, www.medicalnewstoday.com/medicalnews.php?newsid=18777, 11 January 2005.

35. Ibid.

36. "KU Nursing Education and *Cerner* Launch High-Tech Initiative," *Cerner* Corporation news release, 4 March 2002.

37. Ibid.

38. Ibid.

39. Neil Rutkowski, telephone and e-mail correspondence, 2005.

40. Ince, interview, 25 January 2005.

41. Ibid.

42. Ibid.

43. Ibid.

44. Ibid.

45. Rutkowski, telephone and e-mail correspondence.

46. Bill Dwyer, interview by Jeffrey L. Rodengen, audio recording, 9 December 2004, Write Stuff Enterprises.

47. Ibid.

48. Arthur C. Clarke, *Arthur C. Clarke's July 20, 2019: Life in the 21st Century* (New York: MacMillan, 1986), 38-39.

49. Ibid.

50. "Robo Doc: Medicine by 'Extension,'" *USA Today*, 4 August 2004, 8D.

51. Jeff Goldsmith, interview by Antonia Felix, audio recording, 24 January 2005, Write Stuff Enterprises.

52. Jeff Goldsmith, *Digital Medicine: Implications for Healthcare Leaders*, (Chicago: Health Administration Press, 2003), 25-26.

53. Ibid, 18.

54. J. P. Fingado, interview by Jeffrey L. Rodengen, audio recording, 4 November 2004, Write Stuff Enterprises.

55. Goldsmith, 24.

56. Goldsmith, 11.

57. Black, interview, 3 December 2004.

58. James C. Collins and Jerry I. Porras, *Built to Last: Successful Habits of Visionary Companies* (New York: HarperCollins, 1994), 4.

59. Ibid.

60. Ibid, 10.

61. *2003 Annual Report*.

62. Devanny, interview.

63. Mike Herman, interview by Jeffrey L. Rodengen, audio recording, 8 February 2005, Write Stuff Enterprises.

64. Nancy-Ann DeParle, e-mail correspondence, 2005.

Chapter Eight Sidebar:
Cerner Doctrine Physician Services

1. Neal Patterson, "2004 Shareholders Letter," *2004 Annual Report, Cerner* Corporation.

2. John Dragovits, interview by Jeffrey L. Rodengen, audio recording, 11 August 2004, Write Stuff Enterprises.

3. Townsend, interview, 23 August 2005.

Chapter Eight Sidebar:
Cerner Doctrine Implementation

1. "*Cerner*'s Approach to Event-Based Implementations," *Cerner* Corporation document, 5.

INDEX

Page numbers in italics indicate photographs.

Frist, Bill, 144
Fujitsu, 135–136
Fulks, Phil, 49

G

Gavin, Jan, 74–75
Gaylord Palms Resort &
    Convention Center
    (Orlando, Florida), 63
General Data, 63
General Electric (GE)
    Medical Systems, 83
    Mednet project, 24
    PACS, 88
General Hospital (Grey Nuns)
    of Edmonton (Alberta,
    Canada), 89
General Laboratory solutions,
    41
*Genome: The Autobiography of
    a Species in 23 Chapters*
    (Ridley), 126
Gephart, Richard, 144
Germany, 136
Getting Started, 60
Giglio, Chris, 166
global marketplace expansion,
    81–83, *82*, 85, *130*, *139*
    Asia, 132
    Australia, 68, 131
    Canada, 89, 131
    Germany, 132–133
    India, outsourcing,
        136–137
    Middle East, 132
    restructuring to
        accommodate, 139–141
    United Kingdom, 63,
        131–132, *134*
Goldsmith, Jeff, 167
Good Morning America, 26
Gorup, Paul, *15*, *52*, *118*
    Arthur Andersen &
        Company, 14–15
    BDS, launching of, 123
    on *Cerner*'s goals, 87, 98
    education of, 18
    on IT use in healthcare,
        24–25
    on knowledge-based
        solutions, 100
    as Lighthouse architect, 152
    PGI roles of, 29

return of, 123, 126
Gould Evans Goodman
    Associates, 69
Granger, Richard, 63
Grant County, Oklahoma, 16,
    16
Grid systems, 142

H

Hallmark, 58
Hanf, Tom, 110
Hart, David, 89
Harvard Business School, 40
Harvard Medical School, 91
*Healthcare Computing &
    Communications*, 43,
    45, 90
healthcare debate, 145–146
Healthcare Information and
    Management Systems
    Society (HIMSS)
    conference (San Diego),
    129
*Healthcare Information
    Management Systems*,
    27
health care information
    technology (HCIT), 98
Health Care International, Ltd.,
    (Clydebank, Scotland),
    131
Health Facts, 100
Health Midwest, 123
Health Network Architecture
    (HNA), 29, *29*, 30,
    31–32, 35, *35*, 38, 45,
    67, 83
HealthSentry, 103, *103*
Heeren, Andy, 66
Herman, Mike, 50, 52, 155
Hermann Memorial Hospital
    (Houston), 119
Hiawatha Broadband, 146
HNA *Millennium*, 92, *114*, *116*
    cost effectiveness of, 116
    development/testing, 117
    earnings/stocks, effect on,
        113, 119–120, 128–129
    first conversion, 116, 119
    lawsuits, by shareholders,
        128
    planning stage, 109–111
    portfolio, *143*

security features, 114–115
server crashes, system for
    alerting, 117, 119
success of, 128–129
Tablerock, 61, 110, 111
three-tier system, 114
user-friendly features, 114,
    116
Web-based element,
    116–117
wireless technology, 115
Hodes, Matt, 78, 110
Hoffman, Chuck, 17
Holden, Bob, 70, 71
Hollerith, Herman, 23
Hollerith Tabulating Machine,
    22, 23
home healthcare solutions, 103
HomeWorks, 103
Hospital Corporation of
    America (HCA), 45
Hospital Information System
    (HIS), 23
"How to Raise Venture Capital"
    (INC magazine seminar),
    40
H&R Block, 15, 21, 29
Hull, Carol, 121, 122
Human Leukocyte Antigen
    (HLA), *44*, 45
Hurricane Katrina, 81

I

IBM (International Business
    Machines), 18, 21, 23,
    26, 55–56, 63
Idstein, Germany, 136
IDX Systems Corporation, 136
Illig, Cliff, *13*, *15*, *52*, *111*, *118*
    Arthur Andersen &
        Company, 14–15, 17, 18
    on assets, 65, 68
    as Boy Scout/Eagle Scout,
        17
    "The *Cerner* Approach"
        session, 59
    on creating workforce for
        the future, 14
    education of, 17
    on IPO, 71–72
    on Kauffman, 50
    on logo, 120
    on *MedNet*, 89–90